SUTURE LIKE A SURGEON

A doctor's guide to surgical knots and suturing techniques used in the departments of surgery, emergency medicine, and family medicine

M. Mastenbjörk M.D.
S. Meloni M.D.

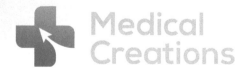

Contents

INTRODUCTION

The word 'suture' refers to the use of a thread-like material to either approximate tissues together, or ligate (seal off) blood vessels. Suturing is a technique that has been practiced for centuries. The first reference to suturing goes back to 3000 BC, and can be found in ancient Egyptian literature. Several materials have been used over the years, including hemp, cotton, and silk. Similarly, needles have also been made of several different materials – bone, silver, bronze, and copper.

Over the years, both the materials used for suturing and techniques have undergone extensive amount of refinement. Suturing techniques today are under sterile, aseptic conditions, and with the use of well-crafted instruments. However, certain principles have remained same over the years, and these are essential for the success and maintenance of tissue integrity.

Most students (and even some residents) assume that the purpose of suturing is to hold incisions together. While this is true, suturing is also useful for a variety of other purposes. Some common applications of suturing techniques are given below:

- ○ To close incisions, allowing primary healing.
- ○ To approximate wound margins after raising a flap or biopsy, allowing secondary healing.
- ○ To promote hemostasis by closing bleeding wound edges.
- ○ To ligate blood vessels.

- ○ To approximate ends of blood vessels (called anastomosis), allowing blood to be re-routed to different areas. One common example of this is the cardiac bypass surgery.
- ○ To repair severed nerves and tendons.
- ○ To temporarily anchor tissues and retract them during surgery, improving access and visibility.

The process of suturing, on the surface, appears to be a simple affair and is generally left to the junior most residents or surgical interns at the end of surgery. However, suturing can also be the most critical stage of surgery. If suturing is not carried properly, a host of postoperative complications can result. These include wound breakdown, incisional hernia, improper healing and scarring, postoperative bleeding, and wound infection. Therefore, it is imperative that students train themselves with skills necessary to carry out the suturing process.

This suturing manual gives you an insight into basics of the suturing process. The first part of the manual will cover the armamentarium required, indications, and basic principles of suturing techniques. The next part will discuss knot tying, different kinds of sutures, and their applications. The last section will also discuss wound care before and after the suturing process.

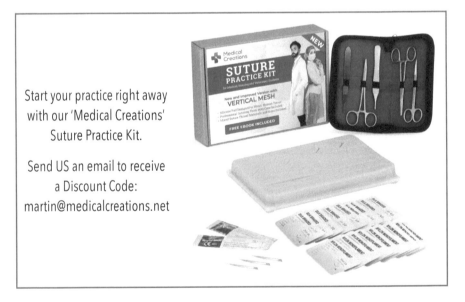

Start your practice right away with our 'Medical Creations' Suture Practice Kit.

Send US an email to receive a Discount Code:
martin@medicalcreations.net

CHAPTER 1

Armamentarium

For successful suturing, two materials are required —surgical needle and suture material. These can be manipulated by a hand-held instrument, namely the needle holder. A few other instruments that come in handy are the tissue holding forceps that helps to stabilize the tissue being sutured, and a pair of scissors for cutting the sutures. Each of these is described in detail in the subsequent sections.

SUTURE NEEDLES

Surgical needles are basically used to carry the suture material into the tissue. They pierce the skin or deeper layers, and transfer the material mounted on them through the tissues. The ideal needle should possess the following properties:

- Be rigid enough to resist distortion.
- Be flexible enough to bend rather than break off.
- Be sharp enough to penetrate tissues easily.
- Be slim enough to cause minimum tissue trauma.
- Be capable of being held snugly in the needle holder without turning.
- Be capable of being sterilized easily.

Usually, needles are made of surgical grade stainless steel, as this fulfills most of the above properties. A needle has three components —eye, body, and tip.

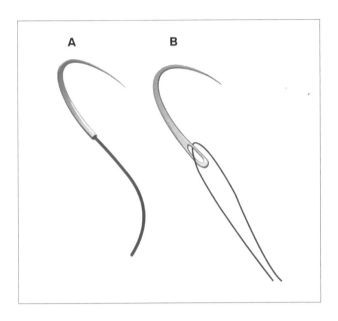

Needle end: This is the portion that contains mounted suture material. The needle can have either an end with an 'eye', through which the suture material is threaded (b), or it can be eyeless. Eyeless needles are also called swaged needles, and the suture material is crimped within the needles (a). Swaged needles produce lesser tissue trauma than needles with eyes, as only one strand of the suture material is pulled through. Needles with eyes carry two strands of material, and possibly a knot through the tissue. This also creates a hole that is wider than the final suture material that remains behind, which can potentially cause leakage and infection. Swaged needles are meant only for single use, and therefore loss of needle sharpness and sterilization do not present a problem. Needles with eyes, however, may be more cost-effective.

In swaged needles, there are two ways of attaching the suture needle to the material – laser drilling, and channel fixation. Laser drilling involves boring a hole into the tail end of the needle, into which the suture is fixed. In channel fixation, a small cut or channel is placed at the needle end for half its thickness, and the material is affixed into this depression.

Needle body: This reflects the shape of the needle. The needle body may either be straight or curved. Curved needles come with different degrees of curvatures, including a half-circle, $1/4^{th}$ circle, $3/4^{th}$ circle, $3/8^{th}$ circle, or $5/8^{th}$ circle. While the $3/8^{th}$ needle is most commonly used for suturing, the other kinds also have certain applications. These have been outlined in Table 1.

TABLE 1. Classification of needles based on body curvature

Type of Needle Body	Applications
Straight needle	Rarely used, when skin closure is done by hand.
Half curved (ski needle)	Laparoscopic surgery.
¼ circle	The shallow curvature makes it convenient for convex surfaces. Used in ophthalmic surgery and microsurgery.
3/8 circle	Most commonly used. Best for superficial and large wounds. It needs a wide arc of rotation, so is not suitable for deep wounds.
½ circle	It is used in confined spaces such as gastrointestinal tract, peritoneum, and respiratory tract.
5/8 circle	Used in deep, confined spaces, does not require much of lateral space for rotation. These include urogenital tract, pelvis, throat, and oral cavity.

Needle tip: It is the point that begins penetration into the tissue. Needle tips may be classified based on their cross-section. The cross-section shape is important as it reflects the ability of the needle to pass through tissues. A sharp cross-section penetrates tissues easily, and is useful for tougher structures. A smooth, round cross-section may be preferable for sift and friable tissues. The different kinds of needle tips and their applications have been outlined in Table 2.

TABLE 2. Classification of needles based on cross-section of the tip

Type of Needle Tip	Cross Section	Applications	Symbol
Round bodied – tapered	Circular, tapers to a point at tip	Muscle, fascia, mucosa, peritoneum, abdominal viscera	

Type of Needle Tip	Cross Section	Applications	Symbol
Blunt round bodied	Circular, rounded tip	Ocular muscle, parenchymatous tissue	
Cutting	Triangle, cutting edge on concave surface	Tough sclerotic tissue, sternum	
Reverse cutting	Reverse triangle, cutting edge on convex surface	Tissues that are tough but can tear, e.g. skin	
Spatula	Trapezoidal	Ophthalmic surgery, microsurgery	

SUTURE MATERIAL

The suture material is of great importance because it is actually going to hold the tissue together during healing phase. This material should therefore have structural integrity, and at the same time, must not cause damage to the tissue. There are several properties that an ideal suture material must possess. These include the following:

- It should be sterile or must be capable of being sterilized without affecting its structural integrity.
- It should be biocompatible, and should not cause tissue reaction or irritation.
- It should be easy to handle.
- It should not fray or break off easily, and allow proper knot security.
- It should have a high tensile strength, maintained during the healing phase.
- Once the healing phase is complete, it should have a suitable absorption profile.

○ It should have antibacterial properties.
○ It should be cost-effective.

Unfortunately, the ideal suture material does not exist at present, and most commonly available materials lack one or more of the above characteristics. Therefore, the surgeon must choose the best possible material depending on the tissue to be sutured, anatomical location, and host factors.

Types of Suture Materials

Suture materials can be classified based on their source of origin as natural materials or synthetic materials. Natural suture materials have been largely replaced by synthetic materials now, as synthetic materials produce less amount of tissue reaction, and have more predictable properties such as tensile strength and rate of absorption. However, natural materials are more cost-effective, and are therefore still widely used in places where cost is a major consideration. Natural silk is often used for securing drains.

Based on behavior of the material in the body, suture materials can be further classified as absorbable and non-absorbable materials.

Absorbable Materials: Absorbable materials get digested by the body enzymes or by hydrolysis after a specific period of time. The rate of absorption is important for these materials, as the absorption process obviously weakens the structural integrity of the material. Ideally, absorption should start only when the wound has gained adequate tensile strength. Absorption rate can be influenced by the type of material, the area of the body where the suture is placed, and host factors. These sutures are useful when deeper layers of the body are sutured, as suture removal is not possible in these areas. These materials are also used in areas that heal rapidly, such as small bowel anastomosis, urinary tract, and biliary tract.

Non-absorbable Materials: Non-absorbable materials are preferred when long-term tissue support is needed. These materials either need to be removed manually, or get walled off by the body's inflammatory processes. These can be used for superficial wounds, wounds that need to heal slowly such as vascular ligation or anastomoses, and to suture muscle, tendons, fascia, and abdominal wall closure. Non-absorbable materials have been divided into three classes. Class 1 consists of silk, nylon, and polypropylene. Class 2 consists of cotton and linen. Class 3 consists of surgical steel. Table 3 lists examples of the different types of materials.

TABLE 3. Classification of suture materials

Natural		Synthetic	
Absorbable	Non-Absorbable	Absorbable	Non-Absorbable
Catgut	Silk	Polyglactin (Vicryl)	Nylon
Chromic catgut	Linen	Monocryl	Polypropylene (Prolene)
		Polydioxanone (PDS)	

Another method of classifying suture materials is as monofilament materials or multifilament materials. As the name suggests, monofilament suture materials have only a single strand. On the other hand, multifilament materials have several strands that are braided or twisted together. While multifilament materials have the advantage of better structural integrity, they have two disadvantages over monofilaments. Firstly, they cause additional trauma to the tissues through which they pass. Secondly, the added bulk of these materials can harbor micro-organisms, and may incite tissue reactions. Monofilaments are more difficult to handle and have poor knot security, but are associated with lower risk of infection. Silk and vicryl are available as multifilament, while most other materials are monofilament.

Suture Material Sizes

Most commonly available suture materials are available in a variety of sizes. Based on their sizes, they are assigned a number in reverse order. The higher the number of a material is, smaller is the size. Different suture sizes have different applications in surgery. These are summarized in Table 4.

TABLE 4. Sizes of suture materials and their applications

Size of Suture Material	Applications in Surgery
0-0 and 1-0	Closure of abdominal wall and securing drain tubes at the wound site.
2-0 and 3-0	Closure of thick tissues, including skin, fascia, muscles, and tendons.
4-0 and 5-0	Skin closure in esthetic areas including hands, feet, face, and skin closure in pediatric patients.
6-0 and 7-0	Plastic surgery and blood vessel repair.
8-0 to 11-0	Ophthalmic surgery and microsurgery including micro vascular reconstruction.

Characteristics of the Suture Material that can Affect Wound Healing Outcomes:

Since the ideal suture material does not exist, the surgeon must make an informed choice based on the characteristics of each material. The following characteristics can affect the final wound healing outcome, and must be kept in mind:

- **Tensile Strength:** Tensile strength refers to the amount of stress that any suture material can withstand before it breaks. Suture materials are prone to several stresses during suture placement, as well as in the postoperative period, owing to swelling and movement. Apart from the initial tensile strength, the rate at which tensile strength is lost over time is also important, and this must parallel an increase in wound strength. The implantation, knotting, and tying of the suture itself causes a loss in tensile strength. Tensile strength is also lost faster in a wet environment.
- **Plasticity:** Plasticity refers to the ability of a material to stretch to accommodate increase in tissue bulk. This is important as most tissues are prone to swelling after surgical manipulation. Plasticity decreases the incidence of tissue strangulation and the formation of cross hatch marks.

9

- ○ **Elasticity:** Elasticity refers to the ability of a suture material to return to its original length after swelling has subsided. If a material is plastic but not elastic, the sutures may become loose after the swelling subsides. Elastic materials ensure that wound margins remain approximated.
- ○ **Memory:** Memory refers to the tendency of the material to return to its original form and shape after it has been bent or manipulated. A material with high memory may be stiff and difficult to handle. Tying knots with these materials can be challenging as the knot may loosen and affect the suture integrity.
- ○ **Pliability:** Pliability refers to the degree of flexibility and the ease with which a material can be bent. Pliable materials are easier to handle and less prone to breakage than non-pliable materials.
- ○ **Coefficient of Friction:** This refers to the degree of slipperiness of the material. A material that is slippery can be handled better and is not prone to break. Sutures with high coefficient of friction can be difficult to pull through and can traumatize the tissue.
- ○ **Biocompatibility:** All suture materials are foreign bodies and therefore cause tissue reactions to some extent. This is greater with natural and multifilament materials. Most suture materials do not cause allergic reactions. However, chromic acids present in chromic catgut have been found to cause allergic reactions in few patients.
- ○ **Antibacterial Activity:** Suture materials do not have intrinsic antibacterial properties. However, materials coated with antibacterial agents are available. Triclosan has been used for coating monocryl and vicryl, and has been shown to reduce colonization by staphylococcus species.

The above characteristics vary with each suture material. Each material must be chosen for specific indications based on the above characteristics. The characteristics and indications for each kind of suture material have been summarized in Table 5.

TABLE 5. Characteristics of commonly used suture materials

Type of Material	Material	Salient Characteristics	Applications
Absorbable	Catgut-Plain	Maintains tensile strength for 7-10 days. Gets absorbed in 70 days. Produces marked tissue reaction. Both tensile strength and rate of absorption are not predictable.	Not commonly used nowadays.
	Chromic Catgut	Treatment with chromic acid delays absorption which occurs around 90 days. Tensile strength lasts for 0-21 days. Can cause allergic reactions due to chromic acid.	Not commonly used, mainly for closure of mucosal wounds.
	Fast absorbing Catgut	Heat treatment facilitates rapid absorption, usually within 2-4 weeks. Tensile strength lasts for 5-7 days only.	Facial wounds, for securing skin grafts.
	Polyglycolic acid	High tensile strength initially, reduces to half by two weeks, and only 5% remains by four weeks. Absorbed in 90 to 120 days. Easy to handle, good knot security. High coefficient of friction.	Closure of deeper layers.
	Coated Polyglycolic acid	Reduced coefficient of friction, but lesser knot security.	
	Fast absorbing Polyglycolic acid	Tensile strength lasts for 7-10 days. Hydrolyzed by 42 days.	

Type of Material	Material	Salient Characteristics	Applications
Absorbable	Polyglactin 910 (Vicryl)	Easy to handle, good knot security. Tensile strength higher than polyglycolic acid, retains 60% strength at two weeks. Absorbed in 60-90 days Biocompatible, low tissue reaction.	Suturing deep tissues. Can also be used for percutaneous closure.
	Vicryl Rapide	Ionization with gamma radiation speeds its absorption, which occurs in 35 days.	Oral wounds, fast absorption minimize irritation.
	Coated Vicryl	Triclosan coating provides antibacterial activity.	Wounds at increased risk of infection.
	Polydioxanone (PDS)	Lower tensile strength than vicryl and polyglycolic acid, but it lasts longer and retains almost 75% strength at two weeks. Stiff and difficult to handle. Minimal tissue reaction.	Useful in wounds that require prolonged dermal support, which minimizes spreading of scars.
	Poliglecaprone (Monocryl)	Highest tensile strength, which decreases rapidly to only 30% by day 14. Pliable, easy to handle, good knot security.	Useful as buried suture where dermal support is not needed.
	Coated Monocryl	Triclosan coating provides antibacterial action.	Areas more prone to infection
Non-Absorbable	Silk	Excellent handling, high knot security. Low tensile strength. High tissue reactivity.	Securing drains. Temporary stay suture to elevate or retract tissues during surgery.

Type of Material	Material	Salient Characteristics	Applications
Non-Absorbable	Nylon	High tensile strength which reduces marginally over time. Gradually absorbs over several years. Stiff, difficult to handle, can traumatize friable tissues. Low knot security. Low tissue reactivity.	Skin sutures. Buried sutures which require prolonged dermal support.
	Polypropylene (Prolene)	Lower tensile strength than nylon. Extremely low tissue reactivity. Does not resorb at all over time. Stiff material, poor handling and knot security. Low coefficient of friction. High plasticity, and can accommodate swelling.	Skin sutures. Areas where more swelling is anticipated. Buried sutures needing long-term dermal support.

HAND INSTRUMENTS

The needle and suture material need to be controlled and manipulated by certain instruments for placing them into and withdrawing them from the tissue. The most basic instruments needed for suturing include needle holder, tissue forceps, and scissors.

Needle Holder

This instrument is used for holding the needle during suturing. It also assists in placement of the knot in certain techniques. The instrument consists of a locking handle, and a short blunt beak. It is easy to confuse this instrument with a hemostat (or artery forceps), which also has a locking handle. However, the needle holder has a shorter beak. The internal face of the needle holder has cross-hatches and a longitudinal groove in the center, which permits a secure grip on the needle. On the other hand, the hemostat has parallel, horizontal grooves that do not permit a proper grip on the needle. The handle of the needle holder may be short or long. Long handles are useful for suturing at depth. Short handles are useful when delicate, fine suturing is required.

To hold the needle holder properly, follow the steps given below:

1. Insert the thumb and ring finger of your dominant hand into the rings of the needle holder. Do not insert the entire finger; only the distal phalanges must remain inside the ring.
2. The index finger may be used to stabilize the needle holder by placing it over the joint. By doing this, the index finger can control the direction of movement of the needle holder.
3. Grasp the needle within the beaks of the needle holder such that it lies one-third the distance from the eye, and two-thirds from the tip. The needle must be held perpendicular to the beaks.
4. Once the needle has been grasped, press the ratchet lock on the handle to secure it.
5. The needle must be removed from the holder prior to tying the knot.

Another method of holding the needle holder is by 'palming' it. In this method, the thumb and ring fingers do not engage the rings of the needle holder. Instead, the thumb rests on the shaft of the instrument on one side, and the ring finger, along with the middle and little fingers, is wrapped around the instrument shaft on the other side. The thenar eminence is used to control the ratchet lock mechanism of the needle holder.

Tissue Forceps

Tissue forceps are also known as 'pickups'. They are used to grasp or stabilize the wound edges while suturing. While there are many different kinds of tissue forceps, Adson forceps are most commonly used for suturing. The forceps may or may not have small teeth at the tips. Toothed forceps provide a better grip, but at the same time may traumatize delicate tissues. In general, toothed forceps must be used for tough tissues such as fascia or skin, while non-toothed forceps must be used for more delicate tissues such as bowel and blood vessels. The tissue forceps must be held between the thumb and the index and middle fingers, similar to a pen grasp. The tissues must be 'picked' up gently. Never crush the tissues.

Scissors

A pair of scissors is needed to cut the sutures after the knot has been placed. Suture cutting scissors should ideally have short beaks and long handles. Scissors must be held in a similar manner as the needle holder, inserting the thumb and ring fingers into the rings of the handle, and using the index finger for stability. The index finger of opposite hand may be used as a rest if sutures are required to be cut at depth. Remember to always cut with the tips of the scissors rather than the flat end of the blade. This gives more accuracy and can avoid unnecessary trauma to the tissues.

Maintaining Sterility of the Armamentarium

All materials and instruments that are used for suturing must be maintained in sterile conditions, and suturing must be done under aseptic conditions to prevent wound contamination. Different components of the armamentarium may be sterilized by different means.

- Suture Materials and Needles: Swaged needles and materials are usually available in a sterile package. The method used is usually ethylene oxide sterilization, and you will find that each suture pack has a label that confirms that the material is EO-sterile. Eyed needles and running suture materials such as silk must be threaded, prior to sterilization. These are then usually sterilized by autoclaving. Bear in mind that repeated autoclaving can compromise the structural integrity of the suture materials.
- Instruments: Instruments used in suturing, namely the needle holder, toothed forceps, and scissors, are also usually sterilized in an autoclave. The suturing kit must either be packed separately, or as part of the surgical kit prior to autoclaving.

All sterile materials and instruments must be handled only with sterile gloved hands. When the floor nurse dispenses sterile suture material, he/she must peel the unsterile outer covering off carefully, and allow it to drop on to the instrument table.

References:

1. Moy RL, Lee A, Zalka A. Commonly used suture materials in skin surgery. Am Fam Physician. 1991 Dec 1;44(6):2123-8.
2. Chu CC. Classification and general characteristics of suture materials. Wound Closure Biomaterials and Devices. 1997;49.
3. Nelson, WJ. Guide to Suturing: Section IIB Instrumentation. Journal of Oral and Maxillofacial Surgery. 2015;73(8):6-16.

——————— S E L F   A S S E S S M E N T ———————

1. Which of the following suture material sizes is useful in microsurgery?
    a. 2-0
    b. 4-0
    c. 6-0
    d. 10-0

2. Which of the following needle types is suitable for delicate, friable tissue?
    a. Cutting
    b. Reverse cutting
    c. Round body taper
    d. Round body blunt tip

3. Which of the following does not improve the handling characteristics of the suture material?
    a. High coefficient of friction
    b. Low coefficient of friction
    c. Pliability
    d. Flexibility

4. Which of the following properties a material must possess in order to prevent sutures from becoming loose?
   a. Plasticity
   b. Elasticity
   c. Memory
   d. Pliability

5. Which of the following suture materials is not suitable when prolonged dermal support is required?
   a. Nylon
   b. Polypropylene
   c. Poliglecaprone
   d. Polydioxanone

6. Which of the following suture materials is suitable in areas that are prone to develop swelling?
   a. Nylon
   b. Polypropylene
   c. Polydioxanone
   d. Polyglactin

7. Which of the following materials is prone to cause inflammatory reactions?
   a. Polydioxanone
   b. Catgut
   c. Nylon
   d. Polyglycolic acid

8. What is the antimicrobial agent used in coated polyglactin?
   a. Chlorhexidine
   b. Penicillin
   c. Metronidazole
   d. Triclosan

9. Which of the following is the correct method of placing the needle in the needle holder?
   a. At the eye
   b. One-third distance from the eye
   c. Half the distance from the eye
   d. Two-thirds distance from the eye

10. Which of the following suture materials takes the longest time to get absorbed?
    a. Catgut
    b. Polyglycolic acid
    c. Polyglactin
    d. Polydioxanone

CHAPTER 2

Purpose and Basic Principles of Suturing

While suturing is a useful and commonly used surgical technique, it is important to know when exactly sutures are needed and when they can be avoided. This chapter will cover the indications and goals of suturing, and outline the basic principles that need to be followed during the placement of any kind of suture.

Goals of Suturing:

- To approximate two edges of the wound so that they remain in contact with each other and facilitate primary healing.
- To support the wound and provide it with tensile strength until the wound develops its own inherent tensile strength by the healing process.
- To eliminate any dead spaces between wound layers.
- To minimize the risk of bleeding.
- To minimize the risk of infection.

Indications for Placing Sutures

- To close wounds unless contraindicated.
- To secure flaps at the recipient site.
- To repair congenital defects such as cleft lip.
- To ligate and transfix blood vessels in order to achieve hemostasis.
- To join two blood vessels together, for the purpose of directing blood flow to a new anatomical site.

- To repair severed nerves and tendons.
- To secure drains, tracheostomy, nasogastric, and gastrostomy tubes.
- To retract tissues to improve access and visibility.

Contraindications for Sutures

- When the wound is superficial and does not gape.
- Wounds on concave surfaces, such as the nasal alar crease and the preauricular sulcus.
- Wounds that are infected must not be sutured unless the infection has been controlled.

Basic Principles of Suturing

Irrespective of the purpose of suturing, certain basic principles have to be followed while placing a suture. While learning how to suture for the first time as a student, attention is paid carefully to these principles in order to place a secure suture. Over time, these become second nature to most of us.

Principles of using the armamentarium:

- Prior to suturing, ensure that the needle and suture material are being held correctly.
- Hold the needle holder in your dominant hand, as described in the previous chapter, between the thumb and ring fingers.
- Place the needle in the jaws of the needle holder at right angles to it, both vertically and horizontally.
- The needle should be held such that it lies in the holder at a point that is one-third the distance from the end (or eye), and two-thirds from the tip.
- Hold the tissue forceps in your non-dominant hand, using a pen grasp.

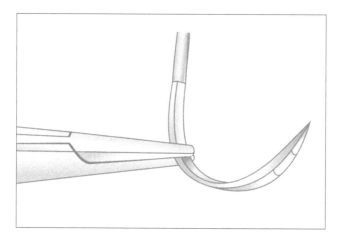

Principles of Taking the 'Bite'

The process of inserting the needle into the tissue and withdrawing it is referred to as a 'bite'. To do this correctly, follow the principles given below.

- ○ Use the tissue forceps to pick up the first wound edge, and evert it gently. This will allow you to visualize the needle as it exits from the opposite side.
- ○ Use the needle to pierce the tissue on one side of the wound. The ideal distance for entering the tissue is around 5mm from the wound edge.
- ○ The needle must enter the tissue at right angles to the wound surface. This allows it to penetrate the wound better, and in an atraumatic fashion.
- ○ Once the needle enters, you must push the needle further into the tissue. While doing so, try to push it following the natural curvature of the needle. This is atraumatic and also provides least resistance from the tissue.
- ○ You will see the needle exit on the inner side of the tissue. Release the needle holder from the 'entering' end of the needle, and use it to instead grasp the 'emerging' end of the needle.
- ○ Pull the needle, with the attached suture material out of the inner wound edge, again following the natural needle curvature.

○ Now the bite must be taken through the second wound edge. Take the bite at the inner edge of the second side (this may vary depending on the technique chosen).

○ Follow the same principles given above for entering and exiting the second wound edge.

○ Remember that the distance of the bites taken on both sides of the wound must be equal. Therefore, if the first bite was taken 5mm from the wound edge, the second bite must also have an exit that is 5mm from the wound edge.

○ Never be tempted to take both bites at once. Taking each bite separately improves the accuracy and saves time in the long run.

○ Similarly, the depth of the bite must be equal on both sides. If the first bite is taken through the skin and subcutaneous tissue, the second bite must be taken from the subcutaneous tissue at the same depth, out through the skin. However, there are certain exceptions to this principle. For instance, a technique referred to as the dermal-subdermal suture technique involves suturing two different layers and therefore different bite depths.

○ Sutures are usually placed from the edge away from you, to the edge towards you. They can also be placed from your dominant side to your non-dominant side. These methods provide the most comfort while suturing. However, the following rules must be kept in mind while taking bites:

- Always suture from movable tissues to fixed tissues.
- Suture from thinner tissues to thicker tissues.
- Suture from deeper tissues to more superficial tissues.

Principles of Placing the Knot

The actual process of knot tying has a separate set of principles, which will be described in a later chapter. However, certain principles need to be kept in mind during this phase of the suturing.

○ Once the needle exits the second wound edge, pull the suture material out of the second wound edge, until only a short length of material remains at the entry point on the first edge.

○ Unclip the needle holder. Setting the tissue forceps aside, collect the long end of the suture material in your non-dominant hand.

○ Knots can be placed either by hand, or using the needle holder. If the needle holder is to be used, grasp it in the dominant hand, and hold it parallel to the wound margin.

○ Place the knot according to the technique desired. The techniques for knot placement are described in the next chapter.

○ The knots must be tight enough to provide adequate security to the suture, and to approximate the wound edges.

○ The knot, however, must not be so tight that it causes strangulation of the wound, or cuts off blood supply.

○ The knot must never lie directly on the wound, as this may interfere with wound healing. It must lie on one side of the wound. If multiple knots are going to be placed, as is the case with interrupted sutures, it is best to place all knots on the same side of the suture line.

Principles of Cutting the Suture

○ Ensure that the scissors used for suture cutting are sharp. Blunt scissors can cause fraying of the suture material, which reduces its integrity for the next suture.

○ Cut off either one or both ends of the suture as desired according to the technique. For running sutures, only the short end must be cut off, while for interrupted sutures, both ends are cut off.

○ For buried sutures placed with absorbable material, cut the sutures as close to the knot as possible. Do not, however, cut right at the knot as this may inadvertently cause knot breakage and compromise the entire suture.

○ For surface sutures that are placed with non-absorbable sutures, do not cut the knot too short. Ideally, at least 5mm of material must be left. This is to facilitate grasping and lifting the material during suture removal.

References

1. Moy RL, Waldman B, Hein DW. A review of sutures and suturing techniques. The Journal of dermatologic surgery and oncology. 1992 Sep;18(9):785-95.
2. Brandt MT, Jenkins WS. Suturing principles for the dentoalveolar surgeon. Dental Clinics. 2012 Jan 1;56(1):281-303.
3. Clark A. Understanding the principles of suturing minor skin lesions. Nursing Standard. 2004;16(1):33-6.

———————— S E L F   A S S E S S M E N T ————————

1. At which point must the needle be held in the needle holder?
    a. 2/3 distance from eye
    b. 2/3 distance from end
    c. Half the distance from eye and end
    d. 1/3 distance from eye

2. In which of the following situations is suturing contraindicated?
    a. Repairing cleft lip
    b. Closing wounds at nasal alar crease
    c. Securing drains
    d. Repairing nerves

3. Which of the following is the correct method of suturing?
    a. Fixed to movable tissue
    b. Superficial to deep tissue
    c. Movable to fixed tissue
    d. Thick to thin tissue

4. What is the ideal distance of taking a bite form the wound edge?
   a. 2 mm
   b. 5 mm
   c. 10 mm
   d. 3 mm

5. How should the suture needle enter and exit the tissue?
   a. In a single straight line
   b. Along the curvature of the needle
   c. Along the contour of the wound
   d. Parallel to the wound

CHAPTER 3

Surgical Knots

Knots are tied at the end of every suture technique, in order to secure the suture in place. Some physicians describe the knot as the 'weakest' link. It, therefore, follows that integrity of the entire suture depends on integrity of the knot. A knot that is not secure can have devastating consequences, from tissue breakdown to severe hemorrhage from a slipped ligature.

Before getting into the various kinds of suture techniques, the student must become proficient in tying different kinds of knots. Knots may be tied either by hand, or by using an instrument. Hand knots can be placed with either both hands or using a single hand.

ANATOMY OF THE KNOT

Irrespective of the method used, each knot basically consists of two kinds of loops. The first loop is called the approximation loop. The integrity of the suture rests on this loop. This loop must be placed in a way that, when tightened, the two edges of the wound are approximated. All additional loops are referred to as securing loops. They provide additional security to the knot.

PROPERTIES OF AN IDEAL KNOT

An ideal knot should possess both the following features:

○ **Loop Security:** This refers to the ability to maintain tightness in the suture while the knot is being tied. Loop security is only influenced by the knot tying technique. Improperly tied knots may be loose and may have low loop security. To achieve maximum loop security, the suture material must be held taut between each throw.

○ **Knot Security:** This refers to the integrity of the final knot. Several factors affect the knot security. These are as follows:

■ Structural Configuration of the Knot: The square knot, which has throws in opposite directions, has more knot security than the granny's knot, which has throws in the same direction.

■ Type of Suture Material: Suture materials with low 'memory' and coefficient of friction tend to have better knot security. Memory refers to the tendency of suture materials to get back to their original shape and form. If a material has high coefficient of friction, the integrity of the material, and therefore knot security can be compromised.

■ Suture End Length: After tying, a suture end length of at least 3mm must be left to optimize knot security.

■ Number of Throws: Certain materials require more throws to secure them. For materials such as nylon, polydioxanone, and polyglactin, at least three to five throws are recommended for optimum knot security. Continuous or running sutures must also be secured with more number of throws.

■ Wound Environment: A fatty environment may compromise knot security, and this should be counterbalanced by more number of throws.

■ Suture Diameter: Knot security increases with increase in suture diameter.

PRINCIPLES OF KNOT TYING

With all the techniques of knot tying, certain basic principles need to be followed. These are outlined below:

- ○ Choose the simplest knot that is indicated under the circumstances. A properly tied knot will remain secure irrespective of the type.
- ○ Avoid a 'sawing' motion during knot tying. This causes unnecessary friction between strands of the material, which may weaken its integrity and cause it to break.
- ○ Avoid crushing the material with the needle holder or tissue holding forceps, which can cause weakening of the material. Only the free ends must be grasped using instruments. Avoid excessive tension and pulling on the material. This can again cause the material to break.
- ○ After placing the first throw or first loop, maintain firm traction on the free end of the material. This will ensure that the knot becomes tight.
- ○ During the final throw, pull the free ends in a horizontal direction to allow the knot to tighten.
- ○ While placing each throw, pull both the free ends in opposite directions – usually one end towards you and the other away from you. This direction must always be reversed in the subsequent throw. When both ends are being pulled, try to maintain uniform rate and tension at each end.
- ○ The final knot must be as small as possible. Extra throws must be used when indicated to add to the security of the knot. On the other hand, there are more chances for a foreign body reaction if the knot is too bulky. Bulky knots placed at deeper layers can also interfere with closure of more superficial layers.
- ○ Above all, once the final knot is placed, it must be ensured that the knot does not slip. If the knot does not appear to be secure, it is better to redo it rather than running the risk of wound breakdown or ligature slippage during the postoperative period.

TYPES OF KNOTS

There are several different methods of tying a knot. A student learning the art of suturing must become proficient in all these types, and must learn to apply the right kind of knot in a given situation. The following section describes in detail the various steps that are used for each kind of surgical knot.

Square Knot

The square knot is a robust, sturdy knot that is most widely used by all surgeons. This is usually placed by hand, and, when an instrument is used, it is commonly referred to as the reef knot.

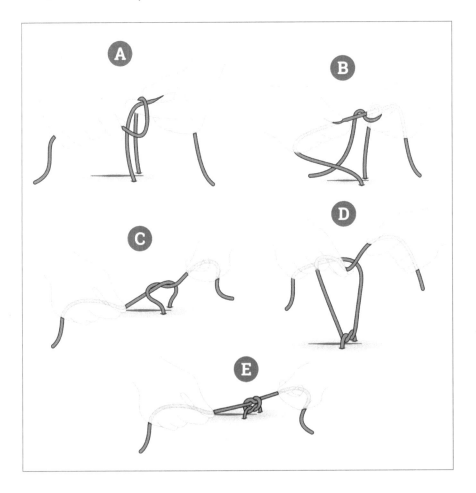

1. Pass the suture material beneath the vessel.
2. Hold the material with both your hands. Keep the left hand away from your body and your right hand close to your body.
3. Pinch the material between the thumb and index finger of the left hand. The longer end of the material must loop around the index finger, go under the vessel, and the other end must be pinched between the thumb and index fingers of the right hand. **Fig. A: First throw.**
4. Cross the material held in your right hand over the index finger of your left. Now this material must be grasped between the thumb and index finger of the left hand, and released by the right hand. A loop will be formed, being held taut by the left index finger.
5. Use your right hand to push the material (which you just transferred) behind the left index finger, through the loop forwards, and out. **Fig. B: Pushing out the first loop.**
6. Using your right hand, pull the material out of the loop, and away from you. Pull the other end towards you. This completes the first half hitch of the square knot. **Fig. C: Tightening the first knot.**
7. For the second half hitch, loop the material held in your right hand over your left thumb, and under it. **Fig. D: Second throw.**
8. Remove your thumb and draw the free ends tight, with your left hand away from you, and right hand towards you. **Fig. E: Final knot.**

This knot must be practiced widely by students. Improper tying of the knot may cause it to turn into a granny knot (described in a following section). This is not desirable because it is much less stable and has a tendency to slip. Another disadvantage of this knot is that even the same operator tends to tie this knot using different amounts of tension. Therefore, if two square knots are placed adjacent to each other by an inexperienced surgeon, the wound may gape slightly because of differing amounts of tension in the two square knots.

Surgeon's Knot

The surgeon's knot is most commonly used when wounds are closed under tension. This knot involves the use of additional 'throws' or loops, which provide greater security to the knot and prevent slippage.

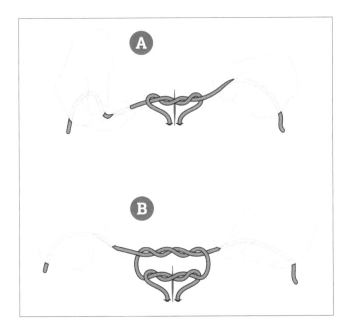

1. Pass the suture material beneath the vessel.
2. Hold the material between both hands, with your right hand near you and your left hand away from you. Pinch the material between the thumb and index fingers of both hands.
3. Loop the material held in your right hand over the index finger of the left, and pull the free end under the material stretched between both hands.
4. Repeat the process of looping around the index finger and pulling the free material once again.
5. Tighten the knot by pulling your left hand towards you and right hand away from you. This completes the first throw. **Fig. A: First throw.**
6. For the next throw, loop the material held in your right hand over your left thumb, and use the thumb to push the free end away from you.

7. Repeat the process of looping over your thumb and pushing the material away.

8. Pick the free end up in your right hand and tighten, by pulling your right hand towards you and left hand away from you. This completes the second throw. **Fig. B: Second throw.**

If a wound can be approximated by using a square knot, a surgeon's knot should not be used. This is because this knot is bulkier than a square knot, and therefore has more potential for foreign body entrapment and tissue reactions. Only if the wound edges do not get approximated using a square knot, should the operator consider using a surgeon's knot.

Granny Knot

The granny knot is not commonly used in wound closure because it has a tendency to slip and may not be secure enough. It is rarely used, when manipulation of the knot tightness is desired.

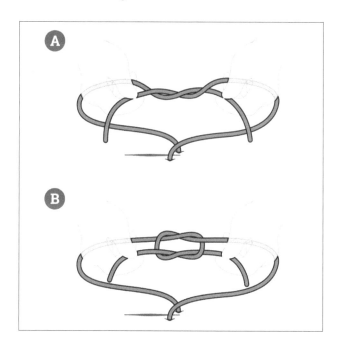

1. Pass the suture material underneath the vessel.

2. Hold a short length of material in each hand, and bring your hands close together.

3. Cross the material in your left hand over the one in your right hand.

4. Push the material which was in the left hand under the right hand material, and bring it towards you and over the right hand material once again. **Fig. A: First throw.**

5. Cross the left hand material over the right again, and loop it under, towards you, and over the right hand material again. **Fig. B: Second throw.**

6. Pull both ends of material tight, in a horizontal direction away from each other.

Slip Knot

The slip knot is useful when the surgeon needs to control the tension under which the wound is closed. The slip knot allows tightening or loosening of the tie, as desired.

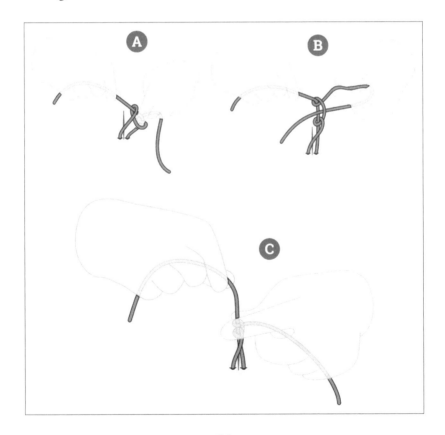

1. Pass the suture material underneath the vessel.
2. The right hand must be kept near you, and use it to hold a shorter length of material between your thumb and index finger.
3. The left hand, which is away from you, must hold a longer length of material between your thumb and middle finger, away from you.
4. While sticking out the index finger of your left hand, pass the material in your right hand around the left index finger and hook it. **Fig. A: First throw.**
5. Draw the left hand material through this hook, and pull it.
6. Repeat the 'hooking' again and pull the knot tight. **Fig. B: Second throw.**
7. You will find that this knot 'slips' easily, and can be pushed down onto the vessel with your left hand, while holding the other end tight with the right hand. **Fig. C: Pushing the knot down.**
8. Usually, a slip knot is completed by applying two reef knots after it for added security. This is an important step, and failure to do so may cause the wound to break down at a subsequent date. This is described in the section below.

Both the granny knot and slip knot are useful for deeper body cavities. In these cases, the knot can be tied at a superficial level and can then be slipped down to the deeper part where it needs to be placed.

Reef Knot

As previously mentioned, this knot is similar to a square knot, but is placed using an instrument. This is commonly used during most suturing techniques for wound closure.

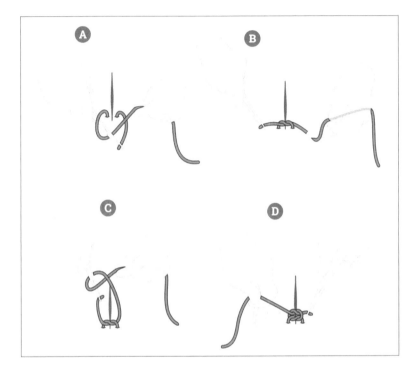

1. Pass the suture material underneath the vessel in such a way that a longer portion is near you and a shorter portion away from you.
2. Take the needle holder in your right hand and grasp the free end of the material that is near you with your left hand.
3. Loop the long end over the needle holder once, in a clockwise direction. **Fig. A: First throw and grasp.**
4. Using the needle holder, grasp the other end of the material and pull it tight, moving the shorter end towards you and longer end away from you. **Fig. B: Tightening.**
5. Loop the longer end of material again over the needle holder, this time in a counter-clockwise direction. **Fig. C: Second throw and grasp.**

6. Grasp the shorter end with the needle holder and pull it tight, moving it away from you, with the long end moving towards you. **Fig. D: Final knot.**

Miller's Knot

The Miller's knot, or its modified version (also called the strangulation knot), is used in the ligation of blood vessels and pedicles. This knot has added security and is very useful while tying off larger pedicles. This can be done using either hand or instrument.

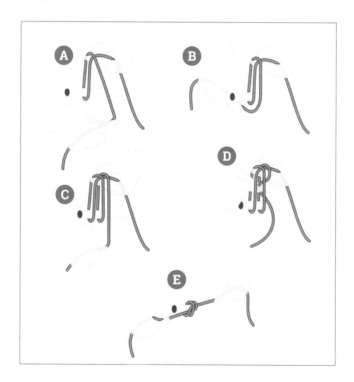

1. Pass the suture material beneath the vessel, keeping your right hand near you and left hand away.
2. Loop the material in your right hand over your left index finger and pinch it. **Fig. A: First throw.**
3. Loop the free end of the same material again around the vessel, around your index finger, and pinch this also, between your left thumb and index finger. **Fig. B: Grasp and pull. Fig. C: Second throw.**

4. Take the needle holder and pass it through the loop, and using this, grasp the free end. **Fig. D: Pulling through the loop.**

5. Pull this tight, bringing your left hand towards you and your right hand away from you. **Fig. E: Final tightening.**

6. The Miller's knot may be tied in another similar way (**MILLER'S 2**). In this, the material must be passed under the vessel and over your left index finger three times, instead of twice **Figs. A to D: Three loops.** The free end of the material must be drawn through the middle loop held by your left hand, and then grasped with your right hand. **Fig. E: Pulling through the middle loop.** Finally, pull tight, moving your right hand away from you and left hand towards you. **Fig. F: Final tightening.**

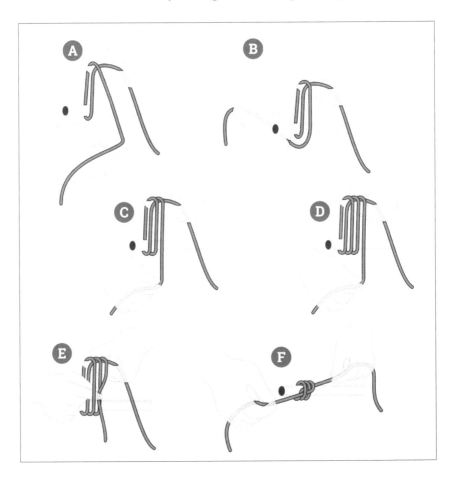

Aberdeen Knot

This knot is used at the end of continuous sutures, using the loose material of the previous section as a loop.

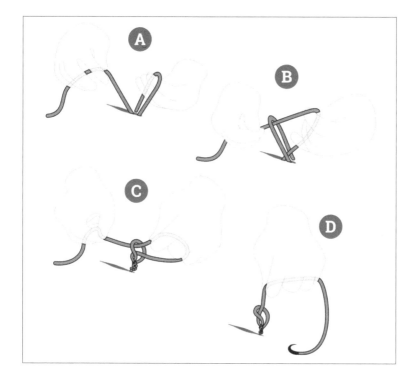

1. The loose loop of the previous section must be held in your left hand, with the long end of the suture material containing the needle in your right hand. **Fig. A: Hold initial loop in one hand.**
2. Using the fingers of your left hand, pull the long end into a loop, and draw it through the existing loop. **Fig. B: Creating the second loop.**
3. The old loop settles down on the wound, and the new loop will now be held in your hand.
4. Repeat the process at least six to eight times for maximum security. **Fig. C: After placing six to eight loops.**
5. At the end, draw the needle itself through the final loop and pull tight. The free end may be cut. **Fig. D: Pulling the needle through the final loop.**

The Aberdeen knot is favored at the end of continuous sutures because it allows the surgeon to place multiple throws without increasing the bulk of the knot too much.

Half Blood Knot

The half blood knot is another knot which involves the use of multiple throws, without resulting in a bulky knot.

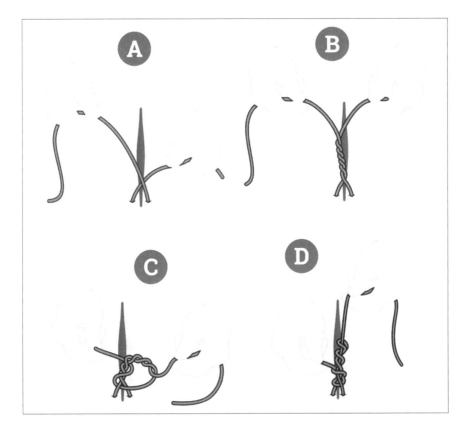

1. Pass the free end of the suture material through the loop formed by the previous section. **Fig. A: Initial loop.**
2. Take the free end of the material, and wind it around itself six to eight times. **Fig. B: Six to eight winds.**
3. Pass the free end of the suture material in the loop formed between the initial loop and the first throw.

4. Now pass the free end of the suture material into the loop formed by the previous step. **Fig. C: Passing through initial and last loop.**
5. Pull the free end tight to secure the knot in place. **Fig. D: Pulling to secure the knot.**

Forwarder Knot

This knot is an example of a self-locking knot. It has added security and does not slip.

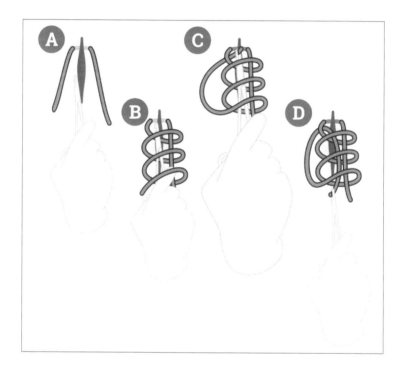

1. To make this knot, first a bite is taken through the tissue.
2. Place the needle holder adjacent to the longer end of the suture material (the end that enters into the tissue). **Fig. A: Place needle holder adjacent to long end.**
3. Wind the free end (the end that exits the tissue, which contains the needle) around both the long end of the material, and the needle holder several times. **Fig. B: Wind free end around long end and needle holder.**

4. Then grasp the free end of the material (with the needle) using the needle holder. **Fig. C: Grasp free end.**
5. Pull the free end with the needle holder tight. The knot will get locked and come to rest on the tissue. **Fig. D: Pull tight.**

Delimar Knot

The Delimar knot is generally used while performing endoscopic procedures. It is especially useful during arthroscopy. The knot is tied using the steps given below:

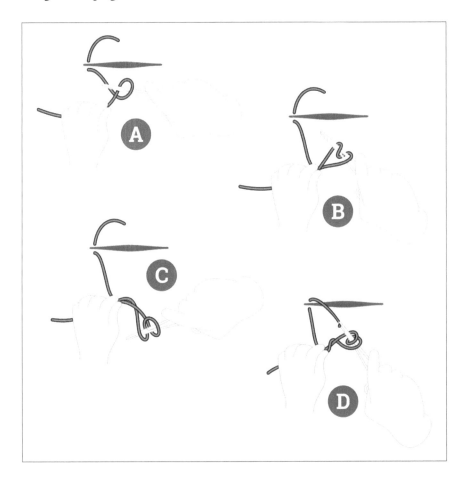

1. Grasp the needle holder in your right hand, and make a loop using the long end of the material adjacent to the needle. **Fig. A: Loop long end.**

2. Take the free end of the material in your left hand. Pass it over the loop made in the previous section, and under the tip of the needle holder. **Fig. B: Pass over previous loop.**
3. Repeat the process with two additional throws. **Fig. C: Additional twist.**
4. Now grasp the free end with the needle holder, pull through the loops, and tighten the knot. **Fig. D: Grasp and pull free end.**

Constrictor Knot

This knot is used for the ligation of blood vessels, and is believed to have more knot security than the Miller's knot. This knot can be tied as follows:

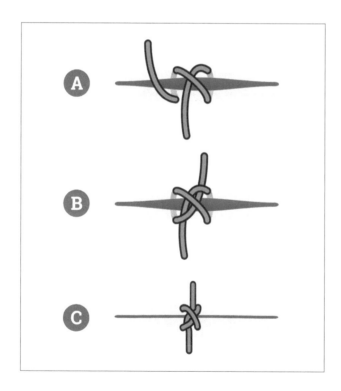

1. Pass the suture material under the blood vessel to be ligated, such that one end lies towards you and the other away from you.
2. Fold the end that lies towards you above the blood vessel and away from you. **Fig. A: Fold near end above and around.**

3. Fold the end that lies away from you over the vessel towards you, and then under the vessel away from you, thus creating a loop. **Fig. B: Fold far end down and under the loop.**
4. Insert the needle holder into this loop.
5. Now turn the free end of the loop behind the other free end of the material, and grasp with the needle holder.
6. Using the needle holder, pull the free ends tight. **Fig. C: Pull tight.**

References

1. Brown RP: Knotting technique and suture materials. Br J Surg 1992;79(5):399-340
2. Silver E, Wu R, Grady J, Song L. Knot Security- How is it Affected by Suture Technique, Material, Size, and Number of Throws? J Oral Maxillofac Surg 2016; 74(7): 1304-1312
3. Richey ML, Rose SC: Assessment of knot security in continuous intradermal wound closures. J Surg Res 2005;123:284-288
4. Taylor H, Grogono AW. The constrictor knot is the best ligature. Ann R Coll Surg Engl. 2014 (96): 101-105

——————— S E L F   A S S E S S M E N T ———————

1. What is the first loop of the knot known as?
   a. Securing loop
   b. Clove hitch
   c. Half hitch
   d. Approximation loop

2. Which of the following factors does not affect knot security?
   a. Surgical technique
   b. Suture material
   c. Suture diameter
   d. Number of throws

3. After placing the final loop, in which direction should the free ends of the suture be pulled in?
   a. Vertical
   b. Horizontal
   c. At an acute angle
   d. At an obtuse angle

4. Which of the following knots is inherently the weakest knot?
   a. Square knot
   b. Surgeon's knot
   c. Granny knot
   d. Reef knot

5. Which of the two following knots are identical?
   a. Reef knot and slip knot
   b. Reef knot and square knot
   c. Reef knot and surgeon's knot
   d. Reef knot and Miller's knot

6. Which of the following knots allows the surgeon control over the tension of the wound?
   a. Slip knot
   b. Square knot
   c. Reef knot
   d. Granny knot

7. Which of the following may be used for ligating bulky blood vessels?
   a. Aberdeen knot
   b. Square knot
   c. Miller's knot
   d. Surgeon's knot

8. Which of the following knots is used for endoscopic suture placement?
   a. Miller's knot
   b. Aberdeen knot
   c. Forwarder knot
   d. Delimar knot

9. Which of the following knots is not suitable for running sutures?
   a. Aberdeen knot
   b. Slip knot
   c. Half blood not
   d. Forwarder knot

10. What is the indication for placing a surgeon's knot?
    a. Wound closure under tension
    b. Ligating bulky blood vessels
    c. Running sutures
    d. Endoscopic suturing

CHAPTER 4

Techniques of Suturing – Basic Sutures and Modifications

All suture techniques are based on four or five basic sutures, which can be modified and applied to several clinical situations. This chapter discusses these basic sutures, and their direct modifications. Beginners must first learn to perform all the basic suturing techniques with skill and speed, before attempting to learn the modifications.

SIMPLE INTERRUPTED SUTURE

Beginners must always start with learning the simple interrupted suture. Once proficient with this method of suturing, you may move on to the other techniques.

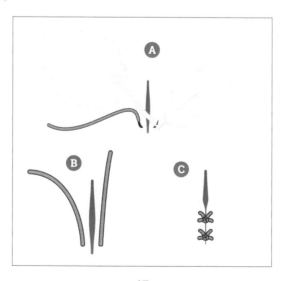

Technique:

1. Always begin the simple interrupted suture at the center of the wound. Once the first stitch is placed, you may place successive stitches at 0.5cm intervals on either side, until you reach the periphery of the wound.
2. Using the tissue forceps, evert the first wound edge, and insert the needle through the superficial surface to the deeper part of the wound edge.
3. Withdraw the needle as it emerges from the deep surface, leaving only a short length (around 2 – 3cm) at the first end.
4. Insert the needle through the deep part of the opposing wound edge. Shift the tissue forceps to this wound edge, while inserting the needle. **Fig. A: Bites.**
5. Withdraw the needle as it emerges from the superficial part, and pull all the material between the two edges taut. Collect the material by swirling it around your non-dominant hand. The initial 2 – 3cm length of material that was left behind should remain as such to be used for knot tying. **Fig. B: Before knot placement.**
6. Place a reef knot as described in the previous section. **Fig. C: Final knot.**
7. Cut both ends of the suture.

Indications and Contraindications:

○ These are the most widely used sutures. They are especially useful in the emergency department for closing lacerations.
○ These are not suitable for placement in deep layers of tissue, or extremely esthetic zones.

Advantages:

○ They are easy to place and can be done by beginners.
○ They provide a high amount of tensile strength to the wound
○ As these sutures are separate from each other, they are able to accommodate tissue swelling efficiently, and thus prevent strangulation of the wound and impairment of blood circulation.

○ The depth and distance of the sutures can be adjusted by the surgeon according to the contour of the wound. This is especially useful in the emergency department where lacerations are rarely neat incisions.

○ If one part of the suture gives way, the other interrupted sutures can still hold the wound edges together. Thus the integrity of the entire suture line is not lost.

Disadvantages:

○ Since each suture requires an individual knot, these are time consuming to place.

○ The sutures tend to leave cross-hatched marks on the skin because of the multiple knots placed. Cross-hatched marks can be avoided by removing the sutures promptly by the fifth day.

Modification: The Simple Buried Suture

This technique is used for closure of deeper wound layers prior to skin closure. The steps of placing a simple buried suture are as follows:

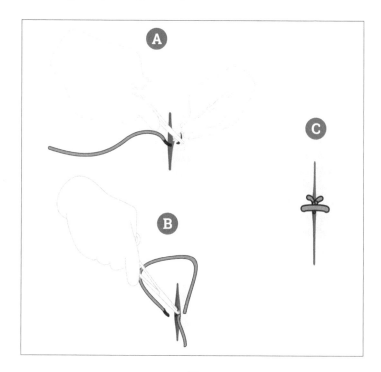

1. The first bite is taken from the deeper part of the wound to the superficial part (unlike the regular interrupted suture, where the first bite goes from superficial to deep). **Fig. A: First bite.**
2. The second bite is taken from the superficial part of the opposing wound edge, to the deep part (again, unlike the regular interrupted suture, which goes from deep to superficial). **Fig. B: Second bite.**
3. Collect the material, as described previously, and place a reef knot.
4. Once the knot is tightened, you will notice that it gets 'buried', that is, the knot tends to lie on the deeper part of the deep layer. This is useful because this knot will not interfere with suture placement on a more superficial layer. **Fig. C: 'Buried' knot.**

Modification: The Simple Interrupted Depth Correcting Suture

This technique is used when there is discrepancy in the depth of the wound between the two edges. This can either be anatomical, or operator-induced by incorrect closure of the deeper layers. The technique for placing this modified suture is as follows:

1. Pierce the superficial surface of the wound edge that is higher than the opposing edge.
2. The needle emerges at the deep surface at a shallow level. For instance, if the superficial surface is the skin, the needle can be allowed to emerge at the dermal-epidermal junction.
3. The needle then enters the deep surface of the opposing wound edge (which is lower in height), not at a corresponding depth, but at a deeper level. In the above example, the needle would enter the deep surface at the dermis or deeper.
4. The needle then emerges on the superficial surface of the opposing wound edge at a similar distance from the wound as the first insertion. Note that only the depth differs, and the distance from the wound does not.
5. A reef knot is then placed. The knot must be of adequate tightness, but not too tight, as this would cause the suture line to look uneven.

SIMPLE RUNNING SUTURE

The simple running suture is a continuous type of suture that can begin at one end of the wound and continue along its length till the other end. No knots are placed in between, and only one knot is placed at the end of the wound length.

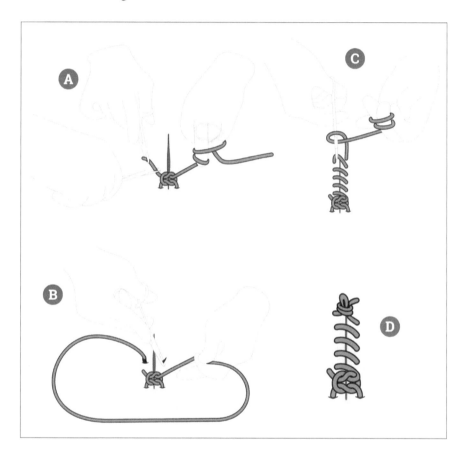

Technique:

1. The first part of the running suture is similar to the interrupted suture.
2. The needle is inserted through the superficial part of one wound edge, taken out through the deep part.

3. The needle is then inserted into the deep part of the opposing wound edge, and taken out through the superficial part.
4. Similar to the interrupted suture, a reef knot is placed.
5. Now, rather than cutting both ends of the suture, only the shorter end is cut and the longer end of the material containing the needle is left intact. **Fig. A: Cutting only the short end.**
6. The needle is brought back to the initial wound edge, and re-inserted from superficial to deep, a few millimeters away from the first insertion.
7. On a parallel point of the opposing wound edge, the needle is inserted and brought out from deep to superficial. **Fig. B: Placing continuous bites.**
8. The process is repeated over and over throughout the wound length.
9. It must be kept in mind that if the bites on opposing sides are directly across each other, the suture will appear diagonal. If the bites on opposing sides are slightly diagonal from each other, the suture tracks appear straight.
10. The last section is left slightly loose to allow for knot placement. **Fig. C: Knot placement.**
11. The reef knot is placed by grasping the 'loose' section of the previous bite instead of a free end. Once the knot is made, both ends can be cut. **Fig. D: Final knot.**

Indications and Contraindications:

○ It is used in long wounds where there is minimum wound tension.
○ Used in securing flaps and skin grafts.
○ It should not be used in wounds that are at increased risk of wound dehiscence.

Advantages:

○ There is less scarring as compared to interrupted sutures because of less number of knots.
○ It is more convenient and much faster to place.

Disadvantages:

- ○ If one part of the suture gives way, the integrity across the entire wound may be lost.
- ○ It is difficult to make fine adjustments along the contours of an irregular wound.

Modification: The Running Locked Suture

Except for one difference, the running locked suture is placed almost exactly the same way as the simple running suture. Each section of the suture is 'locked' by looping the needle through the material. The technique is as follows:

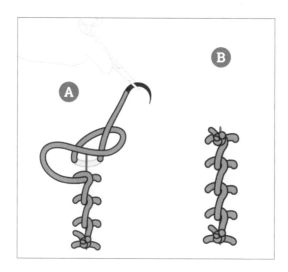

1. The needle is inserted through one wound edge from superficial to deep, and brought out of the wound edge from deep to superficial.
2. A reef knot is placed, and the short end of the suture material is cut.
3. Similar to the simple running suture, the needle is again brought in through the first wound edge and out through the other, few millimeters from the first bites.
4. However, after the needle exits, it must be drawn through the loop of the previous section, thus 'locking' it. **Fig. A: Drawing the needle within the loop.**

5. This process is repeated, and each section is 'locked' with the previous one throughout the length of the wound.
6. The last section, however, must not be locked, and must be left loose to facilitate the placement of a reef knot.
7. After the reef knot is placed, using the 'loop' of the previous bite, the free ends are cut. **Fig. B: Knot placement.**

The running locked suture is generally placed in areas which require increased amount of tensile strength, such as a flap which is being inset into a recipient site, and must establish healing and circulation around its margins. It is also useful in areas where hemostasis is required, or in areas that tend to bleed profusely, such as scalp wounds. However, this suture is not suitable in areas where there is impaired blood circulation, as this suture can cause further strangulation of the tissues.

VERTICAL MATTRESS SUTURE

The vertical mattress suture is also known as the "Donati stitch", named after the Italian surgeon who first described it. This suture provides a more secure method of closing the wound. Moreover, it provides excellent eversion of wound margins as compared to the regular technique.

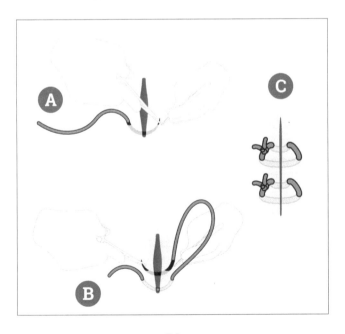

Technique:

1. The needle is inserted from the superficial to deep part of the wound surface, a little away from the wound edge, around 4mm to 8mm.
2. The needle, when emerging from the deep surface, should be at a deeper level, preferably deep to the dermis.
3. The needle then enters the deep part of the wound edge on the opposite side, at the same level, that is, deep to the dermis.
4. The needle emerges on the superficial part of the opposing wound edge, again 4mm to 8mm away from the wound. **Fig. A: Far bites.**
5. The needle is reversed and inserted again into the skin surface on the second side, but closer to the wound edge this time (around 1mm to 2mm from the wound).
6. The needle must emerge on the deep surface more superficial to the previous bites (at or above the dermis).
7. The needle is inserted on the deep surface of the first side, at the same depth.
8. It is brought out on the superficial surface of the first side, again, closer to the wound edge (1mm to 2mm from the wound). **Fig. B: Near bites.**
9. A reef knot is then applied, and the both ends of the suture are cut.
10. This can be repeated throughout the length of the wound. **Fig. C: After knot placement.**

Indications and Contraindications:

○ This technique is applied in areas that are prone to inversion e.g. skin closure after excision of a dermoid cyst. The added eversion provided by even technique results in a flat scar.
○ It is used when closure is done over important anatomical structures, as it provides added resistance against wound breakdown.
○ It is preferably avoided in esthetic areas, because there is high risk of suture marks forming.

Advantages:

- ○ It produces significant wound eversion.
- ○ It tends to reduce dead spaces within the wound.
- ○ It minimizes tension across the wound edges, and provides added tensile strength and support to the wound.

Disadvantages:

- ○ Since this suture has two entry points and two exit points, the risk of cross hatching is greater than even the interrupted suture.
- ○ This technique requires paying great attention to ensure that the four bites are symmetrical. If this is not done, an unesthetic 'shelf' may form on one side of the suture line.

Modification: The Running Vertical Mattress Suture

This combines the advantages of the vertical mattress suture with the running suture, and offers a quick method for close approximation of wound edges with eversion. This technique is performed as follows:

The traditional vertical mattress suture is placed, according to the steps described above. A reef knot is tied.

Instead of cutting both ends of the suture material, only the short end is cut, and the long end with the needle is preserved for the running suture. The technique is performed as follows:

1. The needle is inserted into the superficial part of the wound edge, 4mm to 8mm from the wound, but a little horizontally further along the wound length.
2. It is brought out through the deep part and inserted into the corresponding deep part on the opposing edge.
3. The needle is then brought out through the superficial surface of the opposing edge, 4mm to 8mm from the wound.
4. The needle is then reversed, and inserted from superficial to deep on the second edge, this time 1mm to 2mm from the wound.
5. The needle is inserted from deep to superficial on the opposite side, again 1mm to 2mm from the wound.

6. The needle is once again shifted horizontally along the wound length, to take a bite 4mm to 8mm from the wound.
7. The process is repeated, with two sets of bites (4mm to 8mm, and 1mm to 2mm) at each level, across the length of the wound,
8. Once the end of the wound is reached, a reef knot is placed using the loose loop of the previous section. Both ends of the suture material are then cut.

Modification: Pulley Suture

The pulley suture was designed to reduce the tension across the bites on either side of the suture line. This would reduce the amount of cross-hatching and tissue strangulation that develops. This is placed as follows:

1. The steps used in placing the pulley suture are almost identical to the vertical mattress suture except for the final step.
2. Prior to placing a knot on the first wound edge, the needle is crossed over to the second wound edge, and is looped through the vertical suture 'line' that has formed at this edge.
3. The needle is then crossed back to the first wound edge, and the reef knot is placed before both suture ends are cut.

Modification: Far and Near Suture:

This modification of the vertical mattress suture is basically a modification of the pulley stitch. This technique is done to expand the tissue, when the wound is being closed under tension. The following steps must be followed for placing far and near suture:

1. The first wound edge must be grasped and everted using tissue forceps.
2. The needle is inserted through the superficial part of skin and through the dermis 4mm to 6mm from the wound edge (this is referred to as the far suture bite).
3. The needle is pulled through the deep part of the wound, that is the dermis, and then inserted into the deep part of the opposing side (the side near the operator), at the same depth.

4. The needle is withdrawn through the superficial part of the opposing edge, this time 2mm from the wound edge (This is referred to as the near suture bite).

5. Now, rather than turning the needle back, the needle must be crossed over the wound to the first wound edge.

6. The needle must again pierce the superficial surface of the wound, through the skin and dermis of far edge, but this time, only 2mm from the wound edge. This is again the near suture bite.

7. The needle is pulled out through the dermis and skin of the second edge, 4-6mm from the margin. This is the second far suture bite.

8. The reef knot is then placed, and both the suture ends are cut.

Modification: Half-Buried Vertical Mattress Suture

The main disadvantage of the vertical mattress suture is the cross-hatching, caused due to the four entry points used. This disadvantage is overcome when using the half-buried suture, which eliminates two points on the surface. Therefore, it can be used in areas where esthetics is of concern. This can be placed using the following steps:

1. The needle pierces the superficial part of one wound edge, around 4mm to 6mm from the wound, and exits through the deep surface.

2. On the opposing wound edge, the needle enters the corresponding deep surface. However, it does not exit the superficial surface. Instead, the needle exits again at the deep surface at a slightly higher level.

3. The needle then enters the deep surface of the first wound edge at the same higher level, and exits through the superficial surface, 2mm from the wound.

4. The reef knot is then placed and both suture ends are cut.

5. This method ensures that all marks lie only on one side of the wound, while on the other side, the marks remain invisible.

HORIZONTAL MATTRESS SUTURE

The horizontal mattress suture is another technique that provides pronounced eversion of the wound edge. This technique incorporates much more tissue within a single suture, as compared to the other interrupted sutures, and is therefore often used as an initial suture to hold the wound edges together.

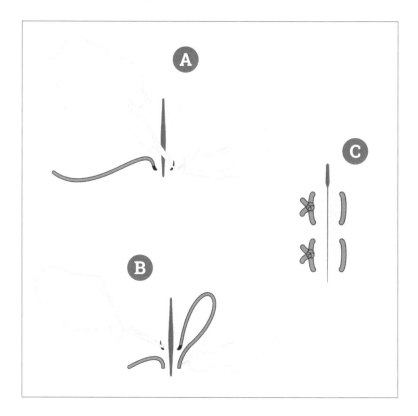

Technique:

1. The needle is inserted into the superficial part of the wound edge. The needle insertion must be at a slightly greater distance from the wound as compared to the interrupted suture, ideally 6mm to 8mm.

2. The needle then exits through the deep part of the wound edge and enters the opposing wound edge at a corresponding level on the deep part.

3. The needle then exits through the superficial part on the opposing edge, again 6mm to 8mm from the wound. **Fig. A: Initial set of bites.**

4. The needle is then reversed and inserted back again into the superficial part of the second wound edge, but a little further down along the length of the wound in a horizontal direction. The distance from the wound must remain the same (6mm to 8mm).

5. The needle exits the deep part of the second wound edge, and enters the corresponding deep part of the first wound edge.

6. The needle exits from the superficial part of the second wound edge, which will be at a short distance horizontally from the very first bite. **Fig. B: Second set of bites.**

7. A reef knot is then placed, and the both ends of the suture are cut. **Fig. C: Knot.**

Indications and Contraindications:

○ Wounds at extremely high risk of wound dehiscence.

○ Used after excision of tissue has been done, when the wound needs to be closed under tension.

○ It is useful as a stay suture, both for retracting tissues, and for approximating tissue edges together during closure using some other technique.

○ Avoid this suture when the tissue has compromised blood supply.

Advantages:

○ Since the sutures are oriented horizontally rather than vertically, it is useful for providing tensile strength to fragile tissues.

○ This technique provides even distribution of tensile strength across the length of the wound.

○ It gives a good amount of wound eversion, allowing the wound to heal faster due to better approximation of edges.

○ It also allows some amount of skin expansion during closure.

Disadvantages:

○ This technique also tends to leave suture marks because, as with vertical mattress sutures, four bites are taken through the tissue.

○ This technique also carries a high risk of tissue strangulation, and can result in necrosis of the wound margins. Cushioning materials, such as bolsters made of gauze, may be placed within the suture material to prevent this from happening.

Modification: The Horizontal Mattress Locking Suture

This technique provides better apposition of the wound edges as compared to the traditional method, and is also easy to remove once the wound is healed. This technique is useful when the tissue is atrophic, as this has less potential for tearing both during suture placement and removal. The method of placement is as follows:

1. The method used is the same as the traditional horizontal mattress suture.
2. Once the needle emerges on the first side, prior to knot placement, the modification is done.
3. The needle is crossed over to the opposite side, and drawn through the horizontal 'loop' formed on the other side of the wound.
4. The needle must be drawn from the side closer to the wound, to the side away from the wound, thus locking the suture.
5. The needle and material are again brought back to the first side, to tie the reef knot. Both ends of the suture are then cut.

Modification: The Running Horizontal Mattress Suture

This technique combines the horizontal mattress and running sutures, and is useful when the eversion obtained with the mattress technique needs to be combined with speed, as is the case for long incisions. This technique is performed as follows:

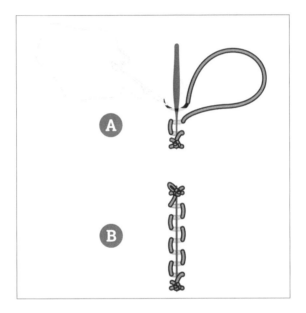

1. A traditional horizontal mattress suture is placed, using the steps given above. The reef knot is tied.
2. Instead of cutting both ends of the suture, only the short end is cut, while the long end containing the needle is retained.
3. The needle is then inserted into the superficial surface of the first wound edge (the edge that contains the knot), horizontally across the knot, at the same distance from the wound.
4. The needle emerges from the deep surface, and pierces the deep surface of the opposing edge at the same level. It emerges from the superficial edge.
5. The needle is reversed, and again used to pierce the superficial surface of the second edge, horizontally a little further away, and it emerges on the deep surface. **Fig. A: Continuous bites.**
6. The needle once again pierces the deep surface of the first edge and emerges through the skin.

7. The needle is once again reversed, and used to pierce the skin, again a little further horizontally. The horizontal movement of the needle continues down the entire length on the wound.

8. Once the end of the wound is reached, a reef knot is tied using the loose loop of the previous section. **Fig. B: Final knot.**

Another modification may be done, combining the two previous modifications. This is referred to as the running locking horizontal mattress suture.

Modification: The Adhesive Strip Bolstered Horizontal Mattress

This method is done for skin that is extremely atrophic, where placement of sutures might cause the skin to tear through. In these cases, placement of surgical adhesive strips can facilitate closure. The wound edges adjacent to the incision must be cleaned and dried to facilitate adhesiveness. The needle bites are then taken through the adhesive strip and the tissue.

Modification: The Half-Buried Horizontal Mattress Suture

The half-buried horizontal mattress suture is more commonly referred to as the 'corner stitch'. This technique is extremely useful for suturing corners of flaps, or the meeting point of incisions that form a 90° angle to each other. The technique is performed as follows:

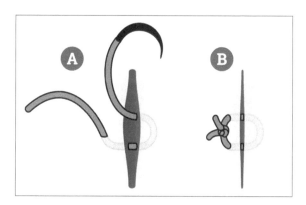

1. An imaginary line must be visualized, bisecting the apex of the triangle vertically. For a beginner learning this technique, it is helpful to actually draw this line on the surface of the skin to establish accuracy.

2. The needle must be inserted on through the superficial skin surface, around 4mm to 6mm above the apex. The point of insertion must be on one side of this line, 2mm to 3mm away from it.

3. The needle is withdrawn through the deep part and taken into the triangular wound area.

4. The flap is everted back using tissue forceps to visualize the deep end.

5. The needle is then inserted on the deep portion of the triangular flap, at a point that parallels the initial entry point.

6. The needle exits through the deep surface of the triangular flap, at a point that is horizontally across the second insertion and diagonally across the first insertion. This would correspond to an area on the other side of the imaginary line, at an equal distance from it. **Fig. A: The 'buried' bite.**

7. The needle is then inserted into the deep surface at a point 4mm to 6mm above the apex, horizontally across the first entry point. The needle exits through the superficial skin surface.

8. A reef knot is then placed. The knot must be tight enough to approximate the tissues so that the corner fits neatly in. Over tightening of the knot may cause the wound edges to buckle and gives an unesthetic result. **Fig. B: Knot placement.**

This technique is most useful when triangular or trapezoidal flaps are raised for access, and are being sutured back in place.

Modification: Buried Horizontal Mattress Suture

This method offers excellent cosmetic results as cross-hatching is avoided. The sutures are placed using the following technique:

1. The first wound edge is everted using the tissue forceps, so that the underlying dermis is visible.

2. The needle is inserted into the dermis around 2mm to 4mm from the suture edge, at an angle that is parallel to the incision line.

3. The needle exits through the same level at the dermis, horizontally across the entry point further along the length of the wound.

4. The opposing tissue edge is then everted to visualize the dermis.

5. The needle is crossed over to the opposite side, and inserted into the dermis at a parallel level to the exit point on the first wound edge.
6. The needle exits through the dermis at a point that is parallel to the initial insertion point on the first wound edge.
7. A reef knot is placed to secure the suture. Both the ends of the suture material are cut.

This technique allows good eversion of the wound edges, but the sutures are invisible. This is useful for suturing narrow wounds, and wounds where it is difficult to insert the needle holder due to lack of space.

Modification: Inverting Horizontal Mattress Suture

As the name suggests, this is a modification of the horizontal mattress suture that produces inversion of the wound edges rather than eversion. This is useful in anatomical areas that are naturally depressed, like skin creases. This technique is carried out as follows:

1. The orientation of the needle is different as compared to other techniques. The needle must be held parallel to the wound edge, rather than at right angles.
2. The needle is inserted from the superficial surface of the wound edge to the deep surface.
3. The needle is then inserted into the deep surface of the same wound edge, a little further along the wound length horizontally.
4. The needle is withdrawn from the superficial surface of the same wound edge, which will be horizontally across the first insertion.
5. The needle is then crossed to the other wound edge, and inserted from the superficial surface parallel to the point at which it just exited.
6. The needle emerges from the deep surface, and it is reinserted into the deep surface of this edge, a little backwards along the length of the wound.
7. The needle emerges from the superficial surface of the second edge. This will correspond to the first insertion point on the opposing edge.
8. A reef knot is then tied, and both suture ends are cut.

FIGURE-OF-8 SUTURE

The figure-of-8 suture is a slightly complicated suture to learn and requires more practice. This technique allows the closure of two or three wound layers in a single suture.

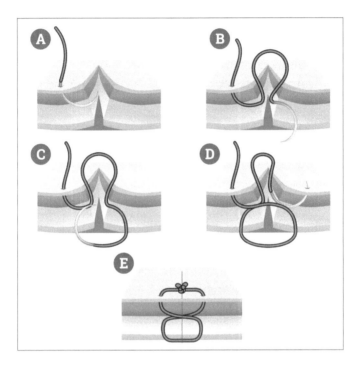

Technique:

1. The needle is inserted through the surface of the skin, and it emerges at the subcutaneous tissue, from which it is withdrawn. **Fig. A: Initial bite.**
2. The second bite is taken through the subcutaneous tissue of the opposite side, at the same level. However, instead of the needle emerging at the skin, the needle is turned downwards to the deeper layer, and is allowed to emerge at the dermis. **Fig. B: Second bite.**
3. The needle is then crossed over to the first side, and it is taken through the dermis at the same level, and out through the subcutaneous tissue. **Fig. C: Third bite.**

4. The needle is once again crossed over to the second side, where it is taken through the dermis to the skin surface. **Fig. D: Fourth bite.**

5. A reef knot is then placed. Both ends of the suture material are cut. **Fig. E: Final knot.**

This is the 'vertical' version of the figure-of-8 suture. There is another version that is placed horizontally. This is similar to the interrupted cruciate suture, which will be discussed in the next section. Surgeons tend to use both these terms interchangeably but it is worth knowing that the 'figure of 8' actually refers to the version described above.

Indications and Contraindications:

○ When you want to suture deep layers but need to remove the suture later on (for instance, when the patient is allergic to resorbable material).

○ For suturing of wounds that have opened up.

○ For wounds that have a round or elliptical contour, or for 'dog-ear' defects.

○ For wounds in which there is a discrepancy in length of the both edges

○ It is best avoided for long wounds, as multiple sutures can be challenging to place.

Advantages:

○ This technique allows the closure of multiple layers at once.

○ Provides good apposition of the wound edges to each other.

○ This technique causes less tissue strangulation, and therefore, less ischemia and necrosis as compared to other sutures, as the tension is distributed across several layers.

Disadvantages:

○ This method is technically challenging as compared to the previous sutures, but can be mastered with practice.

○ Suture removal causes more discomfort to patients as the material has to be pulled out from the deeper layers.

INTERRUPTED CRUCIATE SUTURE/CRUCIATE MATTRESS SUTURE

This suture combines the properties of the simple interrupted suture, the mattress types of sutures, and the running suture.

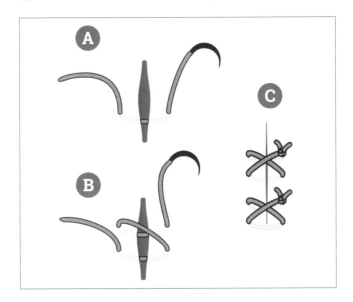

Technique:

1. The needle is inserted through the superficial surface of the wound edge, and is withdrawn through the deep surface.
2. The needle is then inserted into the deep surface of the opposing wound edge at the same point, and is withdrawn through the superficial surface. **Fig. A: Initial bites.**
3. The needle is then crossed back to the first wound edge, and is inserted into the superficial surface at the same distance from the wound edge, but horizontally a little further along the length of the wound.
4. The needle is taken out through the deep surface, and is inserted into the deep surface of the opposing wound edge at the same level.
5. The needle then emerges on the superficial surface of the second wound edge, at a corresponding distance from the first exit bite on this edge. **Fig. B: Second set of bites.**

6. The needle is crossed over to the first side again, and a reef knot is tied such that the knot lies on the first side of the wound.
7. An 'X' is thus formed over the suture line. The process is repeated throughout the length of the wound. **Fig. C: Knot.**

Indications and Contraindications:

○ This is mostly done for the same indications as a simple interrupted suture, except when the wound is longer and the operator wants to save time.

○ It is used when the operator desires a more secure wound placement by tying of multiple knots.

○ It is also useful for minor wounds which are not under tension, such as punch biopsy wounds and tooth extraction sockets.

○ When this technique is used for the ligation of blood vessels, it is sometimes referred to as the 'horizontal' figure-of-8 suture.

○ This is not suitable in areas with compromised blood supply.

Advantages:

○ Can close asymmetrical wounds, such as round or elliptical defects.

○ Provides good approximation of wound edges, and is secure.

Disadvantages:

○ This suture can cause strangulation of tissue if the knots are too tight, leading to wound edge necrosis.

○ This technique does not give perfect esthetics, and is best avoided in esthetic zones.

References:

1. Adams B, Anwar J, Wrone DA, Alam M. Techniques for cutaneous sutured closures: variants and indications. Semin Cutan Med Surg. 2003 Dec. 22(4):306-16
2. Zuber TJ. The mattress sutures: vertical, horizontal and corner stitch. Am Fam Physician. 2002 Dec 15;66(12):2231-6
3. Alam M, Goldberg LH. Utility of fully buried horizontal mattress sutures. J Am Acad Dermatol. 2004 Jan. 50(1):73-6

4. Moody BR, McCarthy JE, Linder J, Hruza GJ. Enhanced cosmetic outcome with running horizontal mattress sutures. Dermatol Surg. 2005 Oct. 31(10):1313-6

5. Lakshmanadoss U, Wong WS, Kutinsky I, Khalid MR, Williamson B, Haines DE. Figure-of-eight suture for venous hemostasis in fully anticoagulated patients after atrial fibrillation catheter ablation. Indian Pacing Electrophysiol J. 2017;17(5):134–139.

SELF ASSESSMENT

1. Which suture technique is commonly used in the emergency department?
   a. Simple interrupted suture
   b. Simple running suture
   c. Horizontal mattress suture
   d. Vertical mattress suture

2. Which suture is also known as the Donati stitch?
   a. Horizontal mattress suture
   b. Vertical mattress suture
   c. Simple running suture
   d. Running locked suture

3. Which of the following sutures involve taking bites at two different depths?
   a. Simple interrupted suture
   b. Simple interrupted depth correcting suture
   c. Simple interrupted buried suture
   d. Cruciate Mattress suture

4. Which modification of the vertical mattress is aimed at preventing cross hatching?
   a. Running vertical mattress suture
   b. Pulley suture
   c. Half-buried vertical mattress suture
   d. Far and near suture

5. Which suture technique is useful for securing the corner of flaps?
   a. Running horizontal mattress suture
   b. Running vertical mattress suture
   c. Half-buried horizontal mattress suture
   d. Half-buried vertical mattress suture

6. Which of the following suture techniques has the least risk of cross-hatching?
   a. Simple interrupted
   b. Simple running
   c. Horizontal mattress
   d. Vertical mattress

7. Which suture technique is useful for skin creases?
   a. Interrupted cruciate suture
   b. Inverting horizontal mattress suture
   c. Figure of eight suture
   d. Buried horizontal mattress suture

8. If a patient is allergic to absorbable sutures, which suture can be ideally placed for the deeper layers?
   a. Interrupted cruciate suture
   b. Inverting horizontal mattress suture
   c. Figure of eight suture
   d. Buried horizontal mattress suture

9. Which suture is useful for closing elliptical wounds?
   a. Interrupted cruciate suture
   b. Inverting horizontal mattress suture
   c. Figure of eight suture
   d. Buried horizontal mattress suture

10. Which of the following techniques is useful when the wound is narrow but deep?
    a. Interrupted cruciate suture
    b. Inverting horizontal mattress suture
    c. Figure of eight suture
    d. Buried horizontal mattress suture

CHAPTER 5

Techniques of Suturing – Advanced Sutures

Advanced suture techniques may not commonly be used in surgery, but they are worth knowing as most of them have their own niche applications. These techniques may either be combinations of various kinds of basic sutures, or may involve a different methodology altogether. This chapter illustrates some of the advanced methods that are commonly practiced by surgeons.

HYBRID SUTURES

Hybrid sutures combine more than one basic type of suturing technique. This offers the advantages of both the techniques. Some examples are given below:

Running Vertical Mattress and Simple Suture:

This method combines the far-near modification of the vertical mattress with the simple running suture. This is useful in delicate tissues where it is desirable to avoid strangulation, but the wound edges must be securely approximated and everted. This technique is performed as follows:

1. The technique begins like a simple running suture.
2. The needle is inserted through the skin of one wound edge, and brought out through the dermis. It is inserted through the dermis of the other wound edge, and brought out through the skin at the same level.

3. A reef knot is tied. The short end alone is cut.

4. The needle is then inserted into the skin immediately near the knot, and brought out diagonally across the wound, well away from the tissue (6mm to 8mm).

5. The needle is then reversed in its holder. It re-enters the skin of the same wound edge at the same level, this time nearer (2mm to 4mm) to the wound margin.

6. It emerges from the dermis, crosses to the dermis of the first edge, and emerges from the skin, again 2mm to 4mm from the wound margin.

7. The needle is then inserted into the second wound edge at the same level, but 6mm to 8mm away from the tissues.

8. It is again directed diagonally, so that it emerges little further along the length of the wound. Now the needle is simply crossed to the opposite side to take a bite similar to a running suture.

9. After this, the far-near, near-far sequence is repeated.

10. The two sutures are alternated till the end of the wound is reached.

11. A reef knot is then tied, using the loose loop of the previous section. Both the suture ends are cut.

Hybrid Mattress Suture:

This suture combines both the horizontal and vertical mattress sutures in a single stitch. It can be used to close epidermal wounds that would normally require a vertical mattress, but just wide enough that a horizontal can close the gap faster. This produces pronounced eversion and good tissue approximation. The technique is performed as follows:

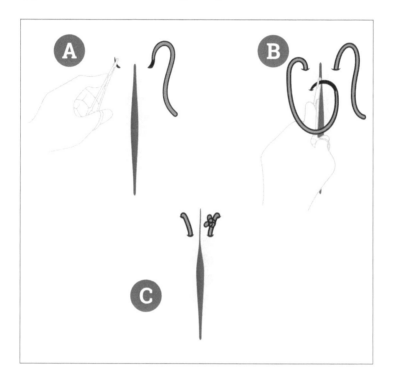

1. The needle is inserted through the skin surface on one wound edge, well away from the wound margin (6mm to 8mm).
2. The needle is taken out through the dermis, and inserted into the dermis at the same level on the opposing wound edge.
3. The needle emerges through the skin on the opposing wound edge 6mm to 8mm from the wound margin. **Fig. A: Initial entry and exit bite.**
4. Now the needle is directed to a point that is nearer to the wound margin (2mm to 4mm away), but also horizontally further along the length of the wound.

5. The needle is inserted into the skin at this point, which leaves a diagonal track of material. **Fig. B: Second entry bite.**
6. This is in contrast to the vertical track seen with the vertical mattress, and horizontal track seen with the horizontal mattress suture.
7. The needle is allowed to emerge from the dermis, and is then inserted into dermis of the first wound edge.
8. The needle is then taken out through the skin of the first edge, at a point that is directly across the previous point of insertion.
9. A reef knot is tied. **Fig. C: After knot placement.**
10. Both short ends are cut. Once the reef knot is tied, it will be noted that another diagonal has formed on this wound edge, and the entire suture has a 'V' shape.

Vertical Mattress Tip Suture:

This suture is a hybrid of the vertical mattress suture and the corner stitch that was described as a modification of the horizontal mattress suture in the previous chapter. This technique is also used to secure corner (or V-shaped) flaps. It is used when there is a risk of the tip getting set deeper than the rest of the flap, as this technique maximizes wound eversion. The technique is performed as follows:

1. The needle is inserted at one of the edges on the concave side of the 'V', around 5mm to 6mm away from the wound margin.
2. The needle emerges at the dermis within the 'V'.
3. The needle then crosses to the convex part of the flap, and pierces the dermis on one side, again 5mm to 6mm from the tip of the apex.
4. It emerges at the dermis on the other side of the apex, at the same level of 5mm to 6mm from the tip.
5. The needle crosses again to the concave part of the flap, and pierces the dermis of the second wound edge.
6. It emerges through the skin, 5mm to 6mm from the wound margin.
7. Now, the needle is reversed in the holder. It pierces the skin of the same wound edge again, this time closer to the margin (2 mm to 3mm).

8. The needle passes from the dermis, to emerge through the dermis within the 'v'.
9. The needle now passes to the dermis on the convex side, and pierces it just 2mm to 3mm from the apex on one side.
10. It emerges at the dermis on the other side of the apex, at the same distance.
11. The needle then pierces the dermis of the very first wound edge, and emerges from the skin 2mm to 3mm from the wound margin.
12. A reef knot is then applied. Both ends of the suture material are cut.

Hybrid Mattress Tip Suture

This suture is a useful technique for securing Y-shaped incisions. This is generally restricted to skin incisions, and the deeper layers are usually closed using other techniques. This technique is performed as follows:

1. The needle is first held perpendicular to the vertical limb of the 'Y'.
2. The needle is inserted from the skin surface around 3 to 4mm from the margin, emerges from the dermis, and pierces the dermis on the other side of the vertical limb.
3. It emerges through the skin at the same level. The needle must not be oriented perpendicular to the diagonal arm of the 'Y' on the side that it has exited.
4. It pierces the skin on the same side, 3mm to 4mm from the diagonal wound edge. It emerges at the dermis in the 'V' component of the 'Y'.
5. Now, similar to the corner suture, the needle is oriented parallel to the dermis.
6. It passes through the dermis on one side of the apex of the opposite edge, and emerges at the same level of the dermis, on the other side of the apex.
7. The needle is now held perpendicular to the diagonal limb of the 'Y' on the other side, and inserted through the dermis.
8. It emerges on the skin of this side, 3mm to 4mm from the margin.
9. A reef knot is applied, using the short end of the material at the beginning of the suture. Both ends of the material are cut.

DERMAL SUTURES/SUBCUTICULAR SUTURES

Dermal suturing is a special technique where sutures do not breach the skin, and remain confined to the dermal layer. This is extremely useful in esthetic zones, as suture tracks do not appear on the skin. The technique is performed as follows:

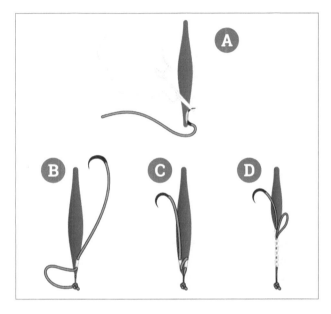

1. The needle must be oriented parallel to the incision throughout this technique.
2. The needle is inserted through the skin surface a few millimeters above the wound apex at one end of the wound. **Fig. A: Bite from wound apex to one side.**
3. The needle is brought out into the dermis, parallel to the incision line. **Fig. B: Bite through dermis on one side.**
4. The needle then crosses to the opposite dermis, and is inserted at the same level, maintaining the parallel orientation. The needle exits from the dermis of the same side, a little further along the length of the wound, maintaining a parallel orientation to the wound. **Fig. C: Bite through dermis on the other side.**
5. The needle again crosses back to the dermis of the first side, and is inserted in a similar parallel direction, to emerge again a little further along the length of the wound on the same side.

6. This process is again repeated, in a continuous fashion on both sides.

7. Once the end of the wound is reached, the needle is brought out through the opposite wound apex. **Fig. D: Closed wound prior to knot placement.**

8. Aberdeen knot, or any knot for a continuous suturing technique is placed. The free end is cut.

9. Aberdeen knot may also be applied at the beginning to prevent the material from going completely into the wound. Alternatively, the material may be secured with surgical tape at both ends, instead of a knot.

PURSE-STRING SUTURE

The purse-string suture is so named because it resembles the string that is pulled to close the mouth of a coin purse. It is useful for round defects, and basically consists of a running suture placed all around the defect. The defect may either be closed off completely, or shrunk to a negligible size using this suture. This is especially useful for sealing off small intestinal defects. This technique is performed as follows:

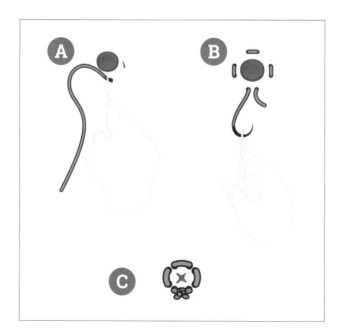

1. The wound edge on the side of the defect that is nearest to the operator is grasped using tissue forceps, and everted.
2. The needle is used to pierce the superficial surface, and is taken out through the deep surface.
3. The needle is again pierced, through the deep surface of the tissue, and is allowed to emerge through the superficial surface, parallel to and a little to the right of the original bite. The distance from the wound should remain the same. **Fig. A: First entry and exit bite.**
4. This procedure is repeated in an anti-clockwise direction around the wound, till the final exit bite is reached, close to the initial point. **Fig. B: Successive bites.**
5. Both ends of the thread are pulled together to close the defect. A reef knot is placed and tightened. Additional throws are required in this technique for added security. A locking knot may be used for better results. **Fig. C: Pulled and closed.**
6. An instrument may be used to invert the edges of the wound while placing the knot, so that the defect is obliterated on pulling the two ends of the suture thread together.

This technique causes the surrounding tissues to pucker, and so must not be used in esthetic areas.

WINCH SUTURE

The winch stitch is designed to close wounds that have excess degree of tension. It is a temporary intraoperative stitch, and its purpose is to hold the tissues in approximation while other sutures are being placed. This technique allows the tissues to draw together by mechanical 'creep' and thus reduces wound tension in the final sutured wound. The technique is performed as follows:

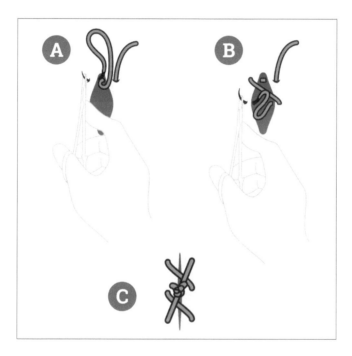

1. The needle pierces the superficial surface of the first wound edge, away from the wound.
2. It emerges from the deep surface, and pierces the deep surface on the opposing edge at the same level. It is then drawn out through the superficial surface. **Fig. A: First bite.**
3. Only a few centimeters of material are left at the initial edge, and this is grasped using a hemostat.
4. The needle is again used to pierce the superficial surface of the first edge, emerges from the deep, and again taken through the opposite side. The process is repeated 4-5 times. **Fig. B: Second bite.**

81

5. The long end of the material is then cut, leaving a few centimeters behind.
6. The hemostat grasping the short end of material is released, and this end is also grasped along with the first end of material. **Fig. C: After successive bites and knot.**

A modification of this technique is referred to as the 'dynamic winch suture'. In this method, the same steps as above are followed. However, the two material ends are held with two different hemostats. Once some amount of tissue creep has occurred, the material is pulled tight with the hemostat, to bring the wound edges closer together. Another hemostat is placed at the junction of the skin and the material, and the hemostat that was pulled is removed. This process is repeated a few times until the wound edges approximate with minimal tension.

CROSS SUTURE

This is a modified simple running suture, used when close approximation of wounds is required. It is also useful for bleeding wound edges, as it can achieve good hemostasis. However, this does not provide added security to the suture, and it can easily come apart even if one part of the material breaks down. This technique is performed as follows:

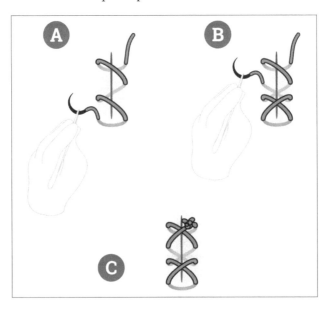

1. The suture starts like a simple running suture.
2. The needle initially enters the skin surface, passes through the deep surface of both edges, and exits out again through the skin surface of the opposing edge.
3. At this point, usually a reef knot would be placed. This is, however, not done, and the short end is instead grasped with a hemostat.
4. The running suture is continued until the entire length of the wound has been covered. **Fig. A: Initial simple running pattern.**
5. The needle is now reversed, and a running suture is continued backwards across the length of the wound.
6. Each bite of the second running phase should be placed in such a way that it forms an 'X' with each bite of the previous running phase. **Fig. B: Running suture continued in backward direction.**
7. Once the beginning of the wound is reached, the hemostat is released and the short end is used to tie a reef knot. **Fig. C: Knot placed.**
8. Both the suture ends are cut. If carried out properly, this technique can give excellent esthetic results.

LEMBERT SUTURE

This is a specialized suture that is used to re-create anatomical structures that are naturally inverted. For instance, the alar crease of the base of nose, and the helical rim of the ear can be sutured using this technique. This is also useful in suturing the gut. This technique encourages inversion of the wound edges. It is performed as follows:

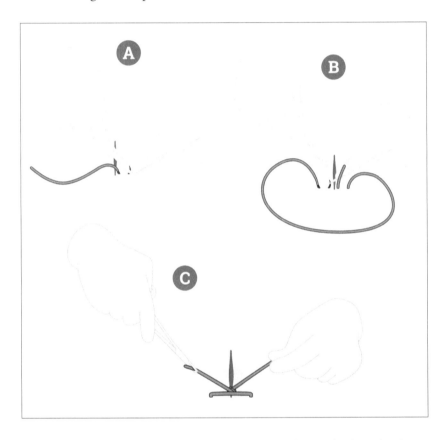

1. The needle is inserted into the deep surface, which is the dermis, and is brought out through the superficial skin surface, a little away from the wound edge. **Fig. A: First bite.**
2. The needle then crosses to the other side and is inserted into the superficial skin surface again, away from the wound edge. It is then brought out through the deep dermis of this side. **Fig. B: Second bite.**

3. A reef knot is placed. The reef knot becomes buried. Both ends of the material are cut. **Fig. C: Knot.**

4. The Lembert suture can also be placed in a running fashion. In this method, only the short end is cut, and the long end with the needle is used to repeat the process by taking alternate bites from the dermis to a point well away from the wound on the skin. This is repeated along the wound length, until the end of the wound is reached. A reef knot is then placed, by grasping the loosened loop of the previous section. Both the free ends are cut.

LATTICE SUTURE

This is another technique that can be used when wounds need to be approximated under significant tension. It is also useful when the tissues are so atrophic that normal sutures cannot hold the tissues together. This technique provides additional reinforcement to the wound and supports tissues better. The technique is performed as follows:

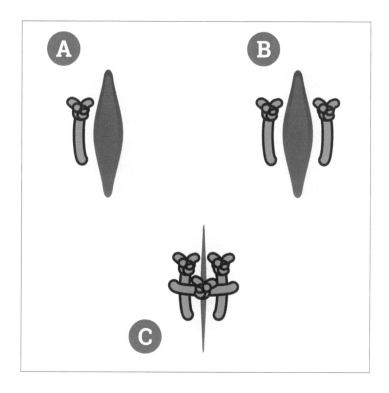

1. Following the steps described in the previous chapter, simple interrupted sutures are placed.
2. However, rather than being placed across the wound, the sutures are placed parallel to the wound or incision, on one side of the wound only. **Fig. A: Interrupted suture parallel to wound.**
3. Sutures must be placed throughout the length of the wound incision.
4. The procedure is repeated on the opposite side of the wound. The sutures on each side of the wound must be in perfect alignment with each other. **Fig. B: Parallel suture on opposite side.**
5. Now, simple interrupted sutures must be placed across the wound.
6. The needle is inserted on the superficial surface of the wound edge on one side, lateral to the previously placed suture, and at the midpoint of the parallel suture.
7. The needle emerges on the deep surface, and crosses to the deep surface of the opposite wound edge.
8. It emerges from the superficial side, again lateral to and at the midpoint of the parallel suture.
9. A reef knot is placed, and both ends are cut. **Fig. C: Interrupted suture across the wound.**

COMBINED VERTICAL MATTRESS DERMAL SUTURE

This is a time saving suture technique than can ideally be applied in deep but narrow wounds. This technique allows closure of multiple layers at the same time, and also allows for eversion of the wound edges. It is similar to the figure-of-8 suture, but is more secure and provides better apposition. The technique is performed as follows:

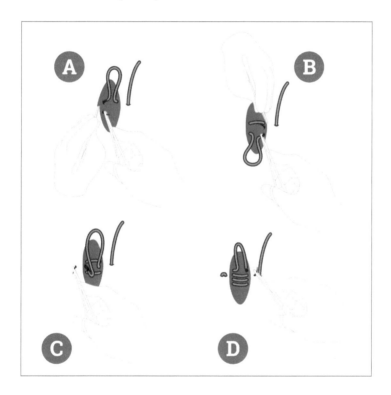

1. The needle is inserted into the skin on one side of the wound edge, 6mm to 8mm away from the wound margin.
2. The needle emerges within the deep dermis on the same side, and is crossed over to pierce the deep dermis at the same level, on the opposing wound edge. **Fig. A: Skin to deep dermis.**
3. The needle is now taken out through the superficial part of the dermis on the second wound edge, and is re-inserted into the superficial part of the dermis, at the same level, on the first wound edge.

87

4. The needle is now made to emerge from the deep part of the dermis on the first edge again. **Fig. B: Deep dermis to deep dermis.**

5. The needle now enters the superficial dermis on the opposing wound edge, and is taken out through the skin of this edge, 6mm to 8mm from the wound margin. **Fig. C: Deep dermis to skin.**

6. The needle is reversed, and inserted back through the skin, 2mm to 4mm from the wound margin.

7. The needle now emerges from the dermal-epidermal junction of this side.

8. The needle is then crossed over, and inserted into the dermal-epidermal junction of the opposite side at the same level.

9. The needle is brought out through the skin, 2mm to 3mm from the wound margin. **Fig. D: Backwards through skin.**

10. A reef knot is then placed. Both ends of the suture are cut.

KESSLER'S LOCKING LOOP

This is a specialized technique that is primarily used for tendon repair. The technique is performed as follows:

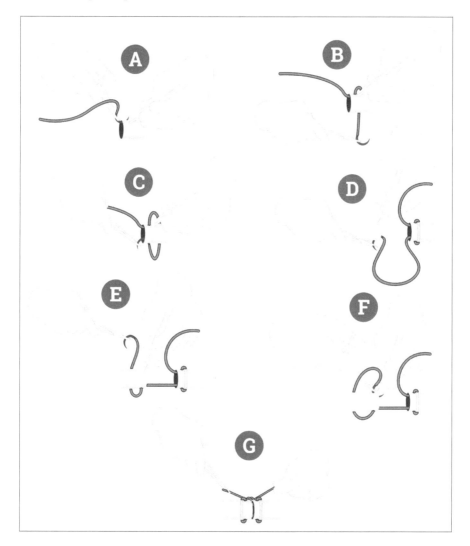

1. The needle is passed from the deep surface of the tendon on one side, to the superficial surface. **Fig. A: First side, first bite.**
2. The needle, with the suture material, is then wound around the tendon, from below, away from the operator, and over the tendon to make a loop. **Fig. B: First side loop.**

3. The needle is now inserted from the superficial part of the tendon to the deep part, thus forming a lock. **Fig. C: First side, second bite.**

4. The needle is then taken to the other part of the severed tendon, and the process is repeated, from deep to superficial. **Fig. D: Second side, first bite.**

5. The needle is again looped around the tendon, this time in the opposite direction (towards the operator). It is again inserted from superficial to deep, and removed. **Fig. E: Second side loop. Fig. F: Second side, second bite.**

6. The free ends on both sides of the tendon are picked up, and a reef knot is applied. **Fig. G: Knot.**

CUSHING SUTURE

This is a continuous inverting suture pattern. It is most useful for suturing the final layer of intestinal incisions. This incision does not penetrate the intestinal lumen, and it only involves the serosa, muscle layer, and submucosa. This technique is performed as follows:

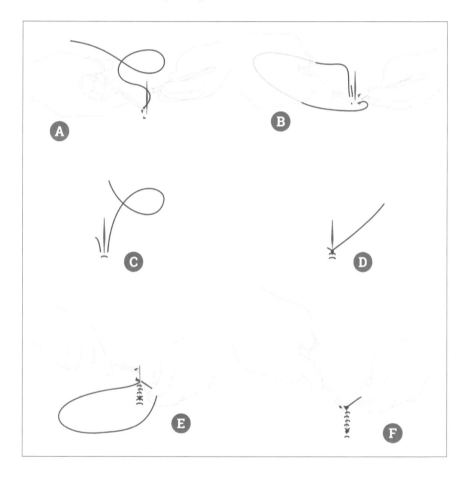

1. The first bite is taken just at or slightly above the apex of the wound, and the suture runs down the length of the wound till the other apex. **Fig. A: First bite.**
2. Initially, this begins like the simple running suture. The needle pierces the superficial surface on one side of the wound, emerges from the deep, penetrates the deep surface on the other side at

91

the same level, and emerges from the superficial surface at the same level. **Fig. B: Second bite. Fig. C: After second bite.**

3. A reef knot is placed, and only the short end is cut. **Fig. D: After reef knot.**

4. The needle must then be oriented parallel to the incision. On one side of the wound edge, a bite is taken through the superficial surface, and it runs through the deep surface to emerge on the superficial surface on the same wound edge, but a little further down the wound length.

5. The needle then crosses to the opposite side, and a similar bite is taken, the entry bite must correspond to the exit bite on the previous side, and the exit bite will be a little further down the wound length.

6. The process is repeated, alternating sides, till the end of the wound is reached. **Fig. E: Continuing along wound length.**

7. A reef knot may be placed using the loose loop of the previous section. It is seen that the wound edges get inverted and the knot gets buried. **Fig. F: Final knot.**

THE RUNNING PLEATED SUTURE

The running pleated suture is used when the two edges of the wound are of unequal length. This often occurs during the insetting of a flap to the recipient site. This technique tends to equalize the length on both sides of the wound, leading to a slightly more esthetic result. The technique is performed as follows:

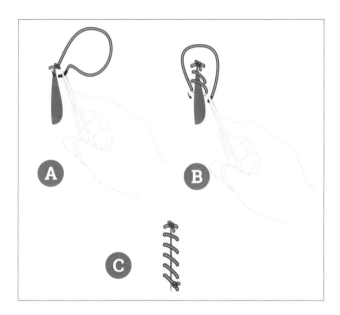

1. The technique begins at the wound apex, where the long and short edges meet.
2. Slightly above the apex, a single interrupted suture is placed, by inserting and withdrawing the needle through the skin, perpendicular to the wound.
3. A reef knot is applied, and only the short end is cut. The needle is then taken to the longer wound edge, a little far away from the interrupted suture (around 6-7mm).
4. A bite is then taken through the longer wound edge, which enters through the skin and emerges relatively superficial on the deep side (at the dermal-epidermal junction). **Fig. A: Excess side—superficial and away from previous.**
5. The needle is then crossed over to the shorter wound edge, and is inserted at a slightly deeper level (deep dermis).

93

6. The needle is taken out through the skin, closer to the initial interrupted suture (around 2-3mm). **Fig. B: Non-excess side— deep and closer bite.**

7. The needle is again crossed over to the long edge, and a wide but superficial bite is taken as before.

8. The needle again crosses to the short edge, where a narrow but deep bite is taken.

9. This process is continued like a running suture, till suturing is completed across the length of the wound.

10. A reef knot is then placed using the loose loop from the previous section. Both the ends are cut. **Fig. C: After wound closure.**

FROST SUTURE

The frost suture is used exclusively after orbital surgery. It is used to maintain the lower eyelid in position, and prevent postoperative ectropion (eversion of the lower eyelid), that can occur due to edema. This technique is performed as follows:

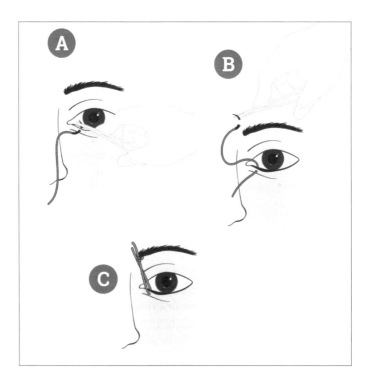

1. The needle is inserted through the skin at the edge of, or just below the medial part of the lower eyelid.
2. The needle emerges at the conjunctival layer of the eyelid. The bite must be narrow, around 3 mm. The operator must be careful to avoid the inferior punctum and canaliculus at all costs. **Fig. A: First bite.**
3. The needle is then inserted and removed through the skin just medial to the eyebrow. **Fig. B: Second bite.**
4. A reef knot is placed and both the ends are cut. **Fig. C: After knot placement.**
5. This suture serves as a sling that suspends the lower eyelid, and prevents it from everting downwards in the postoperative period.
6. The knot at the superior portion can also be replaced with surgical adhesive strips. This allows control over the tightness of the sling in the postoperative period.

THE BOLSTER SUTURE

This suture technique is used to secure a piece of gauze on top of the surgical site. This is useful in skin grafting, where the skin graft needs to adhere firmly to the underlying donor site. This is also useful in providing support to the alar cartilages following rhinoplasty. This technique is performed as follows:

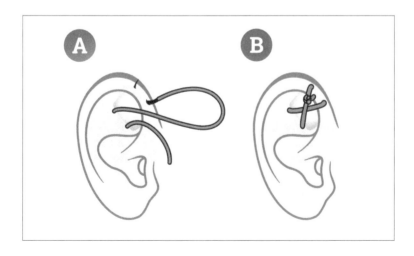

1. A piece of gauze is placed on the skin surface. The operator should place sutures around the piece of gauze, on an imaginary circle.
2. The needle is inserted through the skin at the 6 o'clock position, and is brought out at the 9 o'clock position.
3. The needle is then crossed over horizontally, to the 3 o'clock position.
4. The needle must pierce the skin at this point, and emerge at the 12 o'clock position. **Fig. A: Needle emerging at 12 o'clock.**
5. The needle with the suture material is again crossed over to the 6 o'clock position.
6. A reef knot is placed, and both suture ends are cut.
7. The suture material secures the gauze in place in the shape of an 'X' over it. **Fig. B: Final 'X' shape.**

References:

1. Casparian JM, Monheit GD. Surgical pearl: The winch stitch—a multiple pulley suture. Journal of the American Academy of Dermatology. 2001 Jan 1;44(1):114-6.
2. Yotsumoto T, Mori R, Uchio Y. Optimum locations of the locking loop and knot in tendon sutures based on the locking Kessler method. Journal of orthopaedic Science. 2005 Sep 1;10(5):515.
3. Connolly KL, Albertini JG, Miller CJ, Ozog DM. The suspension (Frost) suture: experience and applications. Dermatologic Surgery. 2015 Mar 1;41(3):406-10.
4. Kouba DJ, Miller SJ. "Running Pleated" Suture Technique Apposes Wound Edges of Unequal Lengths. Dermatologic surgery. 2006 Mar;32(3):411-4.
5. Sadick NS, D'amelio DL, Weinstein C. The modified buried vertical mattress suture: a new technique of buried absorbable wound closure associated with excellent cosmesis for wounds under tension. The Journal of dermatologic surgery and oncology. 1994 Nov;20(11):735-9.

————————— S E L F A S S E S S M E N T —————————

1. Which of the following sutures can be done without leaving any suture marks on the skin surface?
    a. Subcuticular suture
    b. Winch suture
    c. Running pleated suture
    d. Vertical mattress dermal suture

2. Which of the following techniques is ideal for sealing off intestinal defects?
    a. Cross suture
    b. Subcuticular suture
    c. Purse string suture
    d. Kessker's locking loop suture

3. The Frost suture is a specialized suture technique that suspends which of the following structures?
    a. Upper eyelid
    b. Lower eyelid
    c. Suspensory ligament of Lockwood
    d. Nasolacrimal duct

4. Which of the following sutures is useful for insetting flaps into their recipient site?
    a. Lembert's suture
    b. Subcuticular suture
    c. Running pleated suture
    d. Purse string suture

5. Which of the following sutures is used for tendon repair?
    a. Cushing suture
    b. Lembert's suture
    c. Kessler locking loop suture
    d. Running pleated suture

6. Which of the following sutures allows closure of both deep and superficial layers in a single suture?
   a. Running pleated suture
   b. Cross suture
   c. Purse string suture
   d. Vertical mattress dermis suture

7. Which of the following sutures is useful to close wounds that are under a great deal of tension?
   a. Running locked suture
   b. Subcuticular suture
   c. Winch suture
   d. Kessler locking loop suture

8. Which of the following suturing techniques is useful for atrophic wounds?
   a. Cushing suture
   b. Lattice suture
   c. Lembert suture
   d. Winch suture

9. The Cushing suture is just like the simple running suture except for the following important difference
   a. The reef knot is not tied in the beginning
   b. The stitches are oriented parallel to the wound margins
   c. The reef knot is replaced with the Aberdeen knot
   d. Each individual stitch is locked by looping it.

10. This suturing technique provides good esthetics and hemostasis but is not very secure.
    a. Cross suture
    b. Subcuticular suture
    c. Purse string suture
    d. Winch suture

CHAPTER 6

Postoperative Care of the Sutured Wound and Complications

Any sutured wound that is exposed to the external environment requires postoperative care. This obviously does not apply to temporary sutures, such as stay sutures which would have been removed at the end of the surgical procedure. Ligated blood vessels also do not need care once the procedure is over, unless the ligature slips. However, precautions may need to be taken with regard to anastomosed blood vessels.

Postoperative Care of Sutured Incisions and Lacerations

Dressing the Wound:

- ○ Immediately after the final suture is placed, the wound must be dressed to protect it from dust and contamination.
- ○ Never use dry gauze on the wound, as it can adhere to the secretions from the wound, and will be painful to remove at a later date.
- ○ Paraffin gauze, impregnated with antibiotics (such as Sofra-Tulle or Bactigras) are ideal options.
- ○ Alternatively, an antibiotic ointment, such as framycetin cream may be applied on the wound as a thin layer, and gauze can overlie this.
- ○ The medicated gauze is then held in place using surgical tape. Pressure dressings may be used if swelling is anticipated at the wound site.

○ For skin grafts, a gauze bolster may be secured over the graft using tie-over sutures. This will help the graft adhere to the underlying tissue. Further dressing may be done on top of the bolster using paraffin gauze.

Care of the Sutured Wound in the First Few Days:

○ The wound must be kept clean and dry for the first 24 hours.
○ The dressings must be left undisturbed for at least 48 hours, unless there is excessive soakage from blood or inflammatory fluid.
○ After 48 hours, the wound may be gently cleaned with saline or soap and clean water. Antibiotic ointment must be applied periodically.

Removal of Sutures:

Absorbable sutures do not require removal. Non-absorbable sutures need to be removed after a specified period of time, depending on wound healing and the anatomical location. Areas with good blood supply will heal faster, and therefore sutures at these locations can be removed sooner. In general, the following rules are followed for suture removal from various parts of the body:

○ Sutures from the face can be removed in two to three days.
○ Sutures from scalp wounds can be removed in five days.
○ Sutures from the upper limb, groin, and oral cavity can be removed in seven days.
○ Sutures from the abdomen can be removed in ten days.
○ Sutures from the dorsal area of the body, the lower trunk, and limbs can be removed in ten to fourteen days.

The technique to be followed for removal of sutures is as follows:

1. The wound must first be cleaned with saline soaked gauze, to remove friable scar tissue and any encrusted blood.
2. Using the tissue forceps, the knot of the suture must be gently lifted from the surface of the wound.
3. The suture cutting scissors is then used to cut one end of the suture material just below the knot.

4. The forceps is used to pull the knot gently, which allows the suture material to slide out from the tissue completely.
5. The procedure is repeated till all the sutures are removed.
6. For running sutures, cutting only the knot will not suffice. Each loop of the running suture must be lifted and cut, and each section must be removed individually.
7. For removing subcuticular sutures, the knot at the apex on either end must be cut. The suture can be gently withdrawn from within the wound.

Complications

The following complications can occur in a wound that has been sutured.

○ **Wound Infection:**
This occurs when the suture site gets contaminated with micro-organisms. Signs that a wound has been infected include pain, warmth, and redness around the wound site, and unexplained fever. Wound dehiscence may be present with pus discharging from the wound. To manage this, a few sutures must be removed to allow the pus to be evacuated completely. The infected wound must be treated with thorough debridement and antibiotic irrigation. The patient may also be given systemic antibiotics.

○ **Wound Dehiscence:**
Although this can occur as a result of infection, non-infectious causes can also result in wound dehiscence. Inadequate tissue undermining prior to closure, and suturing the wound under tension can lead to dehiscence. If the wound shows no signs of infection, and if less than 24 hours have elapsed since suture placement, re-suturing may be attempted. Otherwise, it is best to let the wound heal by secondary intention without suture placement.

○ **Scarring:**
Esthetic sutures do not leave behind much of a scar. However, if sutures are not removed promptly, or if the suture material has not expanded with wound swelling, 'railroad track' scars may form due to cross-hatching of the suture.

○ **Keloid Formation:**
Keloids are firm masses of scar tissue that proliferate far beyond the boundaries of the original wound margins. This is caused as a hyper-response of the body to wound healing. Although keloids can be surgically removed, they can recur. Steroid injections can help decrease their formation.

○ **Hypertrophic Scar:**
These are similar to keloids, must are not as proliferative, and limit themselves to the wound margins. They are common in joint regions, and unlike keloids, can reduce in size over a period of time. Excision of hypertrophic scars, followed by firm pressure dressings can limit them from forming again.

──────────── S E L F A S S E S S M E N T ────────────

1. Which part of the suture must be cut during suture removal?
   a. The knot
   b. The suture material just below the knot
   c. The suture material just above the knot
   d. The suture material that enters into the tissue

2. Which of the following must not be placed directly on a sutured wound?
   a. Paraffin gauze
   b. Antibiotic impregnated gauze
   c. Dry gauze
   d. Antibiotic ointment

3. When should sutures of the upper limb be removed?
   a. 3 days
   b. 5 days
   c. 7 days
   d. 9 days

4. Which treatment can prevent recurrence of keloids?
   a. Antibiotic cream
   b. Steroid cream
   c. Steroid injections
   d. Surgical excision

5. Which of the following is not a clinical feature of wound infection
   a. Redness of the wound
   b. Pus discharge from the wound
   c. Railroad track formation
   d. Wound dehiscence

ANSWER KEY

CHAPTER 1

1. d
2. d
3. a
4. b
5. c
6. b
7. b
8. d
9. b
10. b

CHAPTER 2

1. d
2. b
3. c
4. b
5. b

CHAPTER 3

1. d
2. a
3. b
4. c
5. b
6. a
7. c
8. d
9. b
10. a

CHAPTER 4

1. a
2. b
3. b
4. c
5. c
6. b
7. b
8. c
9. a
10. d

CHAPTER 5

1. a
2. c
3. b
4. c
5. c
6. d
7. c
8. b
9. b
10. a

CHAPTER 6

1. b
2. c
3. c
4. c
5. c

JOIN OUR COMMUNITY

Medical Creations is an educational company focused on providing study tools for Healthcare students.

You can find all of our products at this link: www.amazon.com/shop/medicalcreations

We want to be as close as possible to our customers, that's why we are active on all the main Social Media platforms.

You can find us here:

Facebook **www.facebook.com/medicalcreations**
Instagram **www.instagram.com/medicalcreationsofficial**
Twitter **www.twitter.com/medicalcreation** (no 's')
Pinterest **www.pinterest.com/medicalcreations**

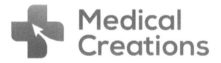

CHECK OUT OUR OTHER BOOKS

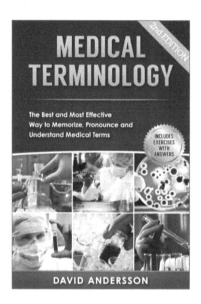

BEST SELLER ON AMAZON:

Medical Terminology:
The Best and Most Effective Way
to Memorize, Pronounce and
Understand Medical Terms

BEST SELLER ON AMAZON:

EKG/ECG Interpretation:
Everything you Need to Know
about the 12-Lead ECG/EKG
Interpretation and How to
Diagnose and Treat Arrhythmias

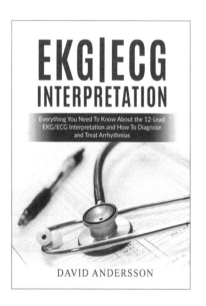

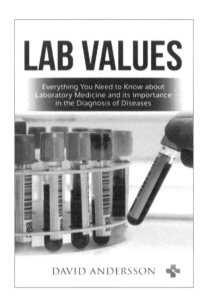

Lab Values: Everything You Need to Know about Laboratory Medicine and its Importance in the Diagnosis of Diseases

Fluids and Electrolytes: A Thorough Guide covering Fluids, Electrolytes and Acid-Base Balance of the Human Body

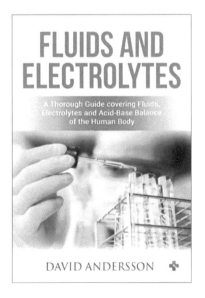